The Massey Lectures Series

The Massey Lectures are co-sponsored by CBC Radio, House of Anansi Press, and Massey College, in the University of Toronto. The series was created in honour of the Right Honourable Vincent Massey, former governor general of Canada, and was inaugurated in 1961 to enable distinguished authorities to communicate the results of original study on subjects of contemporary interest.

This book comprises the 2001 Massey Lectures, "The Cult of Efficiency," broadcast in November 2001 as part of CBC Radio's *Ideas* series. The producer of the series was Philip Coulter; the executive producer was Bernie Lucht.

Janice Gross Stein

Janice Gross Stein is the Harrowston Professor of Conflict Management in the Department of Political Science and the director of the Munk Centre for International Studies at the University of Toronto. She holds the rank of University Professor and is a Fellow of the Royal Society of Canada. She is the author of more than eighty books and articles and the winner of the Edgar Furniss Prize for outstanding contribution to the study of international security and civil-military education. She served as the chair of the Research Advisory Board to the Minister of Foreign Affairs and is currently a member of the International Security Committee of the American Academy of Science and the Committee on International Conflict Resolution of the National Academy of Sciences. She is the mother of two sons and lives in Toronto.

JANICE GROSS STEIN

THE **CULT** OF

EFFICIENCY

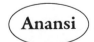

Published in 2001 in Canada and 2002 in the United States by
House of Anansi Press Limited
895 Don Mills Road
400–2 Park Centre
Toronto, ON M3C 1W3
Tel. (416) 445-3333
Fax (416) 445-5967
www.anansi.ca

Distributed in Canada by
General Distribution Services Inc.
325 Humber College Blvd.
Etobicoke, ON M9W 7C3
Tel. (416) 213-1919
Fax (416) 213-1917
Email cservice@genpub.com

Distributed in the United States by
General Distribution Services Inc.
PMB 128, 4500 Witmer Industrial Estates
Niagara Falls, NY 14305-1386
Toll Free Tel. 1-800-805-1083
Toll Free Fax 1-800-481-6207
E-mail gdsinc@genpub.com

CBC logo used by permission

05 04 03 02 01   1 2 3 4 5

NATIONAL LIBRARY OF CANADA CANADIAN CATALOGUING IN PUBLICATION DATA

Stein, Janice Gross
The cult of efficiency

(CBC Massey lectures series)
ISBN 0-88784-668-8

1. Political obligation. 2. Political participation.
3. Educational responsibility. 4. Public health administrations.
5. Responsibility. I. Title. II. Series.

JC329.5.S74 2001   361.613   C2001-901818-5

Cover design: Bill Douglas @ The Bang
Typesetting: Brian Panhuyzen

Printed and bound in Canada

*We acknowledge for their financial support of our publishing
program the Canada Council for the Arts, the Ontario Arts
Council, and the Government of Canada through the Book
Publishing Industry Development Program (BPIDP).*

To my younger sister, Susan,
who taught me early in life that it is better to search
for the hard question than accept the easy answer

Contents

What we do is primarily the result of what we are, and that, therefore the efficiency, or otherwise, of our actions will be determined in the main by what we are: that the habit of Right Thinking must be formed before we can expect Right Doing; that Character and Vision are the Bed-rock of all true Efficiency.

— Lawrence R. Dicksee, *The True Basis of Efficiency*

PREFACE

THIS IS A BOOK ABOUT post-industrial society in the making: the way we organize our lives, what we fear and what we treasure, and how we see the state have altered over the last few decades. I am especially interested in the way we come together in public space and in the language that we use to speak to one another about issues of common concern. My ear has caught more and more public talk about efficiency, accountability, and choice, and less and less about equity and justice. As I have listened, I have often been puzzled. I have also been troubled. How does our public conversation shape the way we as citizens think about our most important shared values? What consequences does it have for the way we construct democratic processes in post-industrial society? A small puzzle has broadened into very large questions.

The Massey Lectures have given me the opportunity to reflect on these questions and to peel away the layers of our public conversation. I began to visit public schools and hospitals to understand how these arguments about efficiency, accountability, and choice come to life in our shared experience as citizens. Public education and health care are among the most basic public goods of concern to citizens everywhere. They matter to me as an individual: my life has been touched by my children's schools and by the health-care system I have turned to at times of greatest personal need. They matter to me not only as an individual, but as a citizen and as a member of the wider community. I use these very local questions as a lens to explore the role of states and markets and the dilemmas of citizenship in post-industrial society.

I could have chosen to listen to conversations about other public goods that we collectively cherish. Our public discussions about water, about the environment, about culture, and even about security raise the same kinds of dilemmas. As I was finishing these lectures, the brutal attacks of terror against New York and Washington created a new sense of vulnerability in North America. Perhaps our sense of vulnerability comes in part from our recognition of how these attacks were carried out: they were perpetrated by a network, the defining form of social organization in the post-industrial age. The new vulnerability that we feel, so familiar to people in many other parts of the world, has pushed to the forefront an ongoing discussion about state and society, about rights and values. We are drawn into a conversation about ourselves and our possibilities, our societies and our commitments. Although the context and the scale are so dramatically different, talk in school corridors and hospital waiting rooms leads us to the same place. It takes us to the deepest and most intractable value conflicts that we face collectively, and to the ways we live with these conflicts in post-industrial society.

Writing these lectures was a voyage of discovery for me, and many people were guides along the way. When Richard Handler, then the executive producer of *Ideas* at the CBC, first asked me to give the Massey Lectures in 2001, I told him that I wanted to write about the dilemmas of post-industrial society. He had expected, I think, an essay focused more sharply on war, or on peace, since I have spent most of my life examining why international conflict is so often intractable, and celebrating those moments in history when we find a way beyond violence. Although he was surprised, his eyes lit up, and in the first early months when I questioned my decision more than once, Richard provided unstinting support and encouragement. That I continued is due in no small measure to him.

I am fortunate to live in a university community, and as I struggled to understand the texture of our public conversation, I was struck again by the generosity of my colleagues and the riches that a citizen of the university enjoys. Carolyn Tuohy, Gina Feldberg, Raisa Deber, and Colleen Flood took time from their busy lives to read successive drafts of the arguments about health care, and answered my persistent questions, sometimes very late at night. I benefited enormously from their knowledge. Ron Manzer offered, as he always does, wise advice on the larger political issues that public education raises. Melissa

Williams accepted no excuses in her response to the last chapter. David Cameron, Ronald Deibert, Louis Pauly, James Orbinski, Michael Trebilcock, Robert Vipond, and Peter Warrian never allowed their friendship to restrain their criticism as they read successive drafts of the whole manuscript. Adele Hurley urged reinterpretation at essential points in the argument. Andrew Goldstein and James Clarke, two young undergraduate students, were superb research assistants. Both became intellectually and personally engaged and dug deep to provide an unending stream of reading.

I imposed on colleagues outside the university as well. Judith Maxwell, in her quietly insistent way, raised the large issues that grew from the small details. Bob Rae suffered through an early draft and insisted on clarity and focus. Philip Siller and Dan Dunsky encouraged me again and again to gnaw at the big questions. Shira Herzog argued with me about the issues and gave the manuscript a final read. Charles Pascal shared his vast experience with me, and my friend, John Fraser, the Master of Massey College, extolled the virtues of tight timelines as I raced against the publishing clock. It is usual now to claim that I and I alone am responsible for all the errors, despite all the help that I received. Here, I accept full responsibility for any errors, and hold my friends and colleagues responsible for whatever light I have been able to shed on some of the challenging dilemmas that we collectively face.

To move from the struggle with ideas to a lucid conversation is no small challenge. Martha Sharpe at Anansi made helpful suggestions and was remarkably patient as I pleaded for more time. Janice Weaver did a superb job of copy-editing the manuscript and Judith Bell provided valuable assistance with the final page proofs. Philip Coulter, my producer at *Ideas*, became a friend as well as a colleague in the months that we worked together on the manuscript. Always encouraging but also demanding, Philip insisted that I could do better, that I could sharpen the arguments. Each round he asked for more, and then more, and I learned from him, often to my surprise, that there was more to give. He is certainly responsible for whatever lucidity and elegance the arguments have.

When I agreed to give the Massey Lectures this year, I made it clear that this was a family project. My husband, Michael, provided unfailing support. He suffered through hours of late night and early morning conversations, gave me reams of material to read, and read drafts of the manuscript again and again. At times, his quizzical look said it all. My two teenage sons, Isaac and Gabriel, were openly pleased that their mother was preoccupied. My niece, Rachel Solomon, endured with grace my endless questions about health care, and Peter Solomon, as always, made intelligent and thoughtful comments about the manuscript.

It is to my sister, Susan Gross Solomon, however, that I owe a special debt of gratitude. She tolerated my early inchoate ramblings and, as the ideas began to take form and shape, quietly but insistently and repeatedly asked the hard questions. With unfailing good humour, she read again and again, and then at times gently and at times not

so gently, moved the conversation. She was never satisfied. It is to her, my oldest and dearest friend, that I
dedicate this book.

Janice Gross Stein
University of Toronto
September 2001

I

THE CULT OF EFFICIENCY

I believe that one ought to have only as much market efficiency as one needs, because everything that we value in human life is within the realm of inefficiency — love, family, attachment, community, culture, old habits, comfortable old shoes.

— Edward Luttwak[1]

The primary function of the Canadian welfare state is not to redistribute wealth — it does almost none of that. Government is involved in the economy because, in many cases, the state is able to deliver goods and services more efficiently than the market.

— Joseph Heath[2]

MY EIGHTY-FIVE-YEAR-OLD mother was hospitalized last year after she shattered her hip. She had been living with me until her accident, but it was now extremely unlikely that she would ever again be able to climb stairs. After the surgery, my sister and I began a frantic search for a suitable place where she could live in safety and with dignity. On the seventh day after the procedure, the discharge coordinator caught me in the hospital corridor; my mother was ready for release, and the coordinator wanted to know what arrangements we had been able to make. I told her that we were doing our best but we would need more time. This was not what she wanted to hear. "Your mother is now a negative statistic for this unit," she said in frustration. "Every additional day that she remains in hospital, she drives our efficiency ratings down."

Never had I thought of my mother as a "negative statistic." Even as I raged at the stinging insult, at the conversion of the whole person into a negative number, I knew that I could not hold the coordinator responsible for anything other than her truthfulness. As a result of a growing insistence on efficiency, her unit had been given seven days to discharge a geriatric patient after a fractured femur. If the patient remained on the floor for eight or ten or thirteen days, the surgical unit became less efficient than the hospital and the government demanded.[3] In our avowedly secular age, the paramount sin is now inefficiency. Dishonesty, unfairness, and injustice — the sins of times past — pale in comparison with the cardinal transgression of inefficiency.

The language of efficiency, or cost-effectiveness, is all around us. We hear it everywhere, in our private lives as well as in public conversation. I recently read an advertisement in a local newspaper for a fully wired kitchen that would allow me to program my microwave and stove from the office simply by flicking a button on my hand-held computer. By the time I reach home, dinner will be ready to eat. The alarm system will disengage as I reach the front door. "How efficient!" the ad proclaims in bold lettering.

But the ad misses, not by accident, I suspect, one crucial piece of information. It does not tell me *at what* this newly wired, very expensive kitchen will be efficient. At improving the quality of my food? At saving time? What, I worried, will I be expected to accomplish with the time saved? Is it legitimate to use the twenty minutes I might gain to read a novel I have been longing to read? Or am I expected to engage in "productive" work in the time that I save? How will this time-saving kitchen improve my satisfaction? My welfare?

The seduction of efficiency is not restricted to the latest advances in labour-saving devices for the beleaguered working mother. The language of efficiency shapes our public as well as our private lives. Those who provide our most important public goods are expected to do so efficiently. Physicians and nurses in the hospital where my mother was treated are expected to work efficiently. So are teachers, governments, and civil servants. They are constantly enjoined to become efficient, to remain efficient, and to improve their efficiency in the safeguarding of the public trust. Efficiency, or cost-effectiveness, has become an end in itself, a value often more important than others. But elevating efficiency, turning it into an end, misuses language, and this has profound consequences for the way we as citizens conceive of public life. When we define efficiency as an end, divorced from its larger purpose, it becomes nothing less than a cult.

A cult is a system of religious worship that engenders almost blind loyalty in its members. Its mystical rites and ceremonies foster in its devotees a sense of belonging and a reverence for core beliefs. Cult members reinforce these beliefs through the incantation of central dogmas. And as the ad for the wired kitchen demonstrates, the invocation of efficiency has approached cult status in our post-industrial age.

I have chosen to examine this cult of efficiency — its origins in thought and in the broader social surround today — in order to try to understand what it reveals as much as what it masks. My conversation in that hospital corridor has stayed with me. I think of it again and again, and it has provoked me to try to understand what efficiency might mean to all of us in the post-industrial age. Writing these lectures has been a voyage of discovery for me as a citizen concerned about the continuing capacity of our governments — and governments around the world, many with far fewer resources than ours — to provide citizens with the fundamental public goods that they need and cherish.

I have chosen to look in particular at how efficiency plays out in our current conversations about public education and health care. Both touch each and every one of us so personally, at so many moments in our lives. Yet education and health care do not meet only personal needs; they are at the core of our relationship as citizens to our governments, and they reflect the ways we think about ourselves as citizens in society.

Health care and education are public as well as private goods, shared by citizens in common space. Economists tell us that public goods, unlike private goods, are not easily divisible. When I breathe clean air, everyone else's air does not become dirtier, but when I eat a slice of my favourite lemon cake, there is less available for others. It is also difficult to exclude people from benefiting from public goods, while it is easier to do so with private goods. Safe streets in the city in which I live are open to everyone, but when I build a fence around my yard, it becomes private space from which I can easily exclude others.

My interest does not lie principally with public education and universal health care, as important as they are, but more generally with public goods in our post-industrial age. And I do not have explicit proposals for reform of the educational and the health-care systems, as urgent as reform is. I leave that to the far more knowledge-able experts with years of experience. However, I do want to listen to the language that we use when we talk about health care and education, and try to decode its meaning.

Although efficiency has been part of our public conversation for centuries, it has never been as prominent in our language as it is today. Why now? Why are we so preoccupied, almost obsessively, with efficiency? What is it about post-industrial society that gives pride of place to efficiency? By following the currents that have come together in our contemporary conversation, we can uncover some of the different political purposes that drive talk about efficiency.

Efficiency, when it is understood correctly as the best possible use of scarce resources to achieve a valued end, is undoubtedly important. Efficiency must always be part of the conversation when resources are not infinite and citizens and governments have important choices to make among competing public goods. It is impossible to dismiss efficiency from our public discussions, and it is a mistake to try. Yet our public conversation about efficiency is misleading.

Efficiency is only one part of a much larger public discussion between citizens and their governments. Efficiency is not an end, but a means to achieve valued ends. It is not a goal, but an instrument to achieve other goals. It is not a value, but a way to achieve other values. It is part of the story but never the whole. When it is used as an end in itself, as a value in its own right, and as the overriding goal of public life, it becomes a cult.

Even when efficiency is used correctly as a means, when it is understood as the most cost-effective way to achieve our goals, much of our public discussion is fuzzy about its purpose. What does effectiveness mean? What, for example, is an effective education? To answer that question, we would first have to discuss the purposes of education, a discussion that is informed by values, and only then could we come to some understanding of the criteria of effectiveness. At times, however, even the mention of effectiveness is absent, and the conversation slides over to focus only on costs. And when the public discussion of efficiency focuses only on costs, the cult becomes even stronger.

Yet the word "efficiency" is not only misused in public conversation as an end rather than a means. Our public conversation is not merely bedevilled by a simple technical error. The cult of efficiency, like other cults, advances political purposes and agendas. In our post-industrial age, efficiency is often a code word for an attack on the sclerotic, unresponsive, and anachronistic state, the detritus of the industrial age that fits poorly with our times. The state is branded as wasteful, and market mechanisms are heralded as the efficient alternative. This argument, we shall see, is based on a fundamental misunderstanding of the importance of the "smart" state in the global, knowledge-based economy.

Our language shapes practice and lives through experience. To understand how the language of efficiency lives, and how the cult of efficiency flourishes, we need to dig down to uncover how the new public markets of education and health care work. Public markets are created when the state no longer directly provides protection to its citizens and uses public money to contract others — public institutions, private firms, and not-for-profit organizations — to supply our most important public goods. What does my mother's story — and the stories of many other patients and students — tell us about public markets for public goods? How do they work? What do they accomplish?

When we look closely at the new public markets in health care and education in chapter 3, we will discover that public markets are not delivering what they promise. They do not provide greater efficiency, but there is a surprising twist: public markets do deliver some unexpected and significant consequences. At times, public markets help in unanticipated ways to build community and to broaden choice among people who historically have had little or none. Most important, public markets are changing the way we see ourselves as citizens, they are changing the face the state shows to its citizens, and they are creating a new and powerful public agenda of accountability.

This agenda of accountability goes to the heart of the relationship between governments and their citizens. It empowers citizens. Citizens in a democratic society have the right to hold their leaders to account for the commitments they make and for the standards they are elected to uphold. The market, we shall see, also uses a language of accountability, but public accountability within the democratic tradition of rights and values has a very different meaning. These two different threads of accountability are spun through the tapestry of our conversation about public goods in the post-industrial age. This conversation is important and worth having. What are those who provide our public goods accountable for? There is more than one answer to this question, and each answer is constructed through larger discussions about the political and social values that are at play in post-industrial society.

The conversation about efficiency, which grows into a richer discussion of accountability, leads us to a deeper debate about values and rights. Running through the talk about education and health care in public markets is a persistent theme of choice as a value and a right. A culture of choice is emerging, nourished by the radical individualism of affluent, comfortable, post-industrial society. The desperately poor and insecure do not often insist on choice as a right. They focus their energy on survival.

The right to choice meets and challenges other deeply embedded rights, and creates tension and contradiction. The sense of openness and possibility that the right to choice promises runs up against the commitments and values that give definition to our society. I want to follow this theme through the current controversies about public education and health care, and explore the contradictions, the dilemmas, and the challenges that the right to choice creates in the way we think about public goods in post-industrial society.

I want to begin by tracing some of the signal moments in thinking about efficiency, moments that have given new meaning to efficiency. An interest in efficiency is not unique to our times. Efficiency has been part of our public conversation for centuries, and it has had different meanings at different times. Which meaning we choose, and why, depends on our larger political purposes and values.

The ancient Greeks, quite naturally, are the starting point, with their understanding of efficiency as one of several instruments that create a virtuous society. For the ancient Greeks, efficiency was a means to higher ends. But efficiency was appropriated and warped into an end when the machine and the factory enabled the industrial revolution; efficiency came to be judged by external measurable standards. It was transformed again as public thinking located efficiency in the rational, bureaucratic state that we came to know throughout the past century. It is no small irony, given our present debates, that a century ago efficiency was embedded within the state as the provider of our most important public goods.

Public discourse turned on its axis again as efficiency became an internal, subjective experience rather than an external standard. This conversation about individual satisfaction, which began more than two hundred years ago among utilitarian thinkers during the industrial revolution, feeds much of our present discussion as citizen-consumers of public goods. It leads away from states toward markets as the preferred providers not only of private goods, but of our most cherished public goods, and toward an emergent culture of choice. This is the defining debate of contemporary post-industrial society, a debate that we cannot fully understand unless we travel through the conversations of the past and follow them into the present.

The Cult of Efficiency

The demand for efficiency is everywhere. We hear it in our private lives, in public life, in wealthy societies, and in the poorest communities. To make certain that I was not imagining that I hear and read about efficiency everywhere, armed with my new — efficient — computer, equipped with a new and more efficient search engine, I searched a widely respected collection of publications for the word "efficiency." In 1990, there were 8,527 references; a decade later, in 2000, there were more than 55,000. Writing about efficiency seems to have increased almost 700 percent in the past decade!

The government of Ontario recently released a report by a task force that was established to evaluate the administrative operations of the province's postsecondary institutions.[4] The report concluded that universities in the province are among those in Canada who spend the least on administration as a proportion of their operating expenses. Universities in Ontario, the report concluded, were generally efficient. Efficient at what, I wondered. The report gave no data on the quality of education these universities provided. It did not ask how well education was being delivered to students in comparison with the costs of administration, so that students — and citizens — in Ontario could make some determination of cost-effectiveness. It did not ask the questions, Efficient at what? For whom? Rather, it valued low central administration costs as an end in itself and defined this as efficiency.

This preoccupation with efficiency as an end is not local and parochial. Far from Canada, in Somalia and Rwanda, in Sierra Leone and Sudan, non-governmental organizations (NGOs) are delivering food, water, and basic health care to millions of displaced people trapped in violent conflict. Almost every recent study of these NGOs calls for greater efficiency in their cost of "doing business." But as one seasoned Canadian observer wryly asked: "Greater than what? Greater than the Ford Motor

Company? Greater than the Japanese Ministry of Transport?"[5] Efficiency clearly takes on different meanings in different spheres of human activity. The yardstick is relative and rooted in context.

The scale of efficiency is one issue. Even more important is the question, Efficient at what? Are NGOs efficient at moving quickly in an emergency, at restoring safe water supplies and clean drinking water, at setting up emergency medical tents, at preventing epidemics, at getting food to those who need it most urgently, at helping wartorn societies recover from violence? Each of these tasks requires different kinds of planning, recruitment of different kinds of professional skills, mobilization of different kinds of resources and different kinds of administrative support. To begin to talk sensibly about the efficiency of NGOs that are assuming the traditional burdens of governments in some of the most dangerous places in the world, we would have to know first what they seek to accomplish. Only then could we evaluate their administrative costs in relation to the difficulty of the challenges they face and the objectives they have set for themselves.

Beyond considering what NGOs seek to accomplish, we would also want to know how well they are accomplishing their goals, how effective they are. If we look only at the administrative costs of an NGO as a proportion of its total spending — as many do — we risk being badly wrong in our analysis. Even more troubling, this kind of analysis of efficiency can seriously distort the agendas of the leaders of NGOs, who may well be tempted to reduce administrative costs regardless of the difficulty of the tasks they are performing. The reduction of administrative costs could actually imperil the capacity of NGOs to work safely and well in very dangerous environments. To ask only "Are NGOs efficient?" without understanding their larger objectives and how well they accomplish these purposes is to truncate an important discussion.

As we would expect, the language of efficiency pervades not only the private and not-for-profit sectors, but the public sector as well. More and more, in the public arena, we see ourselves, and are seen by our leaders and our public institutions, as "consumers."[6] As consumers, we expect that the public services our governments and institutions provide will be delivered efficiently, that we will receive "value for money" — our money. We also expect that like consumers in the marketplace, we will be satisfied with the services that are provided. The language of the market has been gradually extended to the public arena.

Examples abound. Recently, the Senate Committee on Social Affairs urged a shift in emphasis from social expenditure to "social investment."[7] The language of the committee is striking: its members worked to articulate a vision of community and underscored the importance of social justice for the citizens of Canada. Yet they chose, quite deliberately, to use the language of "social investment" to promote values that lie largely outside the parameters of the market. The committee's report was written using the idiom of the entrepreneur and the metaphor of the market.

The same kind of changing vocabulary also appears in recent analyses of the social ties that bind citizens

together and create community. Robert Putnam of
Harvard University has argued that civic engagement —
citizens coming together to participate in public space on
public issues — is a precondition for the creation of
"social capital": the expectations of trust and reciprocity
that are critically important to the effective functioning of
democratic governments.[8] Again, the language is instruc-
tive: the dense network of associational ties that create the
fabric of community becomes social "capital," a resource
that can be depleted or accumulated, invested efficiently
or dissipated. As a measure of the public temper, the
imagery is revealing: the language of efficiency is used to
defend community. It is somehow more acceptable to use
the language of the market than to speak the language of
community and public space.

If the language of efficiency is everywhere — in private, not-for-profit, and public life — efficiency as a
concept is often used in very different ways with very different meanings. Efficiency is, as I've already mentioned,
not a new concept, but dates back to ancient times, before
markets grew parallel to states. Untangling these different meanings through time is helpful in tracing the
different threads that still inform public conversation. I
believe that there are at least three important threads to
follow: efficiency considered objectively as a productive
machine; efficiency considered subjectively as internal
satisfaction; and the promise of markets to deliver efficiency where states have failed. These three threads, I
think, weave the tapestry of our present conversation.

Thinking about Efficiency: The Productive Machine

The modern concept of efficiency developed in the context of the rationalist spirit of the Enlightenment and the bustling commercial activity of eighteenth-century England. Adam Smith used the concept explicitly after he saw a pin being made in a factory. The production of a pin requires about eighteen different operations — such as cutting the wire, grinding the head, and straightening the wire. Smith calculated that if one worker did all these tasks, he could make no more than twenty pins a day. When the tasks were divided among different workers, however, factories could produce about 4,800 pins per worker per day.[9] Smith explained these large gains in efficiency by the division of labour and markets:

> The being of a market first occasioned the division of labour, and the greatness of it is what puts it in one's power to divide it much. A wright in the country is a cartwright, a house carpenter, a square-wright or a cabinet maker, and a carver of wood, each of which in town makes a separate business.[10]

Smith did not worry about the consequences of individual pursuit of self-interest for the collective good.[11] Writing in the early stages of the industrial revolution, he was confident that the invisible hand, working through the market, would harmonize the individual pursuit of self-interest with the collective interest:

It is not from the benevolence of the butcher, the brewer, or
the baker that we expect our dinner, but from their regard
to their self-interests. We address ourselves not to their
humanity but to their self-love, and never talk to them of
our necessities but of their advantage.[12]

Private vices would become public virtues. The individual pursuit of self-interest would collectively control
individual excess and promote the public good.

Developed against the backdrop of the industrial revolution, Adam Smith's thought is a watershed in the
thinking about public goods: public goods could be provided through efficient private exchange in markets.
Efficiency became fully embedded in public consciousness — and discourse — during the industrial revolution
and the automation of work.

Although we associate the concept of efficiency with
the project of modernity and the mechanical age, it was
part of public conversation much earlier. The ancient
Greeks spoke of efficiency, but as a means, not an end, of
politics and society. Long before the industrial revolution,
Plato made what seems at first glance to be an argument
similar to that of Adam Smith about the division of
labour: "More tasks of each kind are accomplished," Plato
argued, "and the work is done better and done more easily, when each man works at the one craft for which
nature fits him."[13] But the differences between the
Platonic analysis of the division of labour and Adam
Smith's are far more important than the similarities. In
Plato's ideal world, deduced through rationality or right

reason, the role of each individual is derived from inherent natural differences that fit each person to specific tasks. The Platonic division of labour is an argument not about individuals engaging in efficient exchange, but rather about the efficient combination and utilization of human resources to approximate the ideal state. Each citizen becomes virtuous by performing the most efficient role in society; society most nearly approaches the ideal type when individuals accept the definition of their proper role as prescribed by those with the highest powers of reason.[14]

In Platonic thinking, the purpose of efficiency is virtue: efficiency is the achievement of virtue by government through reason, and the ends of efficiency are virtue and justice. Embedded in this concept of efficiency produced by the division of labour is a concept of the accountability of citizens to the *polis*, to the political community, and of the *polis* to its citizens. Thinking about efficiency is tied to values — and to accountability. No concept could stand in sharper contrast to the modern cult of efficiency.

The three English words "efficiency," "effectiveness," and "efficacy" all derive from the same Latin verb, *efficere*. It captures all the dimensions of efficiency, bringing together the whole rather than focusing on one part, separate from the larger context. *Efficere* translates from the Latin as "to bring about, to accomplish, to effect." Only in modern times do we separate effectiveness, efficacy, and efficiency, and our public conversation is consequently fractured — and impoverished.

The concept of efficiency changed radically as modern science revolutionized the way we see ourselves, our relationship to nature, and our possibilities.[15] It began in the twelfth century and continued through astronomical thinking in the sixteenth century, when Galileo's examination of time and motion sowed the seed for the idea of the human being as a machine. This picture of the human as machine developed in tandem with the invention and multiplication of machines such as the mechanical clock and the printing press, which had finely measured, standardized, and replaceable parts.

The development and refinement of machines extended the horizon of human possibilities, first to control and then to master nature, and enabled a discussion of efficiency as increasing productivity, as an almost limitless capacity to produce more and more at the same cost. "There is only one efficient speed, *faster*," writes Lewis Mumford in his wonderful analysis of the myth of the machine. "Only one attractive destination, *farther away*; only one desirable size, *bigger*; only one rational quantitative goal, *more*."[16] The mechanical worldview created a language of the measurable, the quantitative, and the productive. Machines became progressively more lifelike and humans became progressively more like machines, culminating, during the industrial revolution, in the new language of the factory. Gradually, this language spilled over into our description of ourselves, our management of our work, and eventually the state itself.

Students of human energy, working early in the nineteenth century, thought of the human machine as superlatively efficient. The German physiologist Edmund Munk argued that the "human motor" was the "most complete dynamic machine" in comparison with other machines; they waste nine-tenths of their heat in the conversion to force, while the body uses only 40 percent of its chemical materials in the production of work.[17] The body was extraordinarily efficient, these nineteenth-century physiologists argued, through the "law of the least effort" — the internal economy of the conversion process within the human body.

Auguste Chauveau, working at the Collège de France, closely examined how human muscles work and developed the "law of the least effort" in physiology. The contracted muscle, he argued, "is the result of a special and absolutely perfect elasticity of the muscles . . . adapted to the functional purposes envisaged and anticipated by muscular work." The principle of efficiency is embedded in the economy of work performed by muscles, so that the "human motor" always chooses "the most economic course."[18]

The language and the imagery of these early physiological studies of human energy are striking. The human body is like a machine, a human motor, but more efficient than any machine that humans had yet made. Inside our bodies, these nineteenth-century physiologists told us, we have an efficient system that converts energy to work. Efficiency is not imposed from outside; it is not alien. We are inherently, innately, superbly efficient. Efficient is what we are; and it is a natural progression from "what we are" to "who we are."

Once we began to think of people as naturally efficient machines, it was not a large step to the science of management, so central to the development of contemporary society. The roots of scientific management can be traced back to the mathematical and technical calculations of mechanical engineers in the nineteenth century. The growing importance of thermodynamic machines in the industrial revolution gave precision to the study of efficiency. Engineers began to use the term "efficiency" to describe the ratio of useless energy to useful energy a machine produces. Drawing on the early laws of physics, they introduced the word "useful" into the vocabulary of efficiency.[19] Embedded within the concept of "usefulness" is a value judgement.

These early studies of the efficiency of machines were paralleled by the analysis of the human machine. The physiologists who studied the efficiency of the human motor at work began the analysis of time and motion. They broke down work into its smallest measurable units by calculating the amount of time, as well as the amount of energy, that each unit of work required. Although their calculations are long outdated, the principles are familiar to students of time management and productivity.

At the beginning of the twentieth century, Frederick Winslow Taylor was the most famous preacher of the new gospel of scientific management in the industrial workplace. He stood, with paper and timepiece in hand, observing workers on the factory floor, fully believing that every act of every worker could be reduced to a mechanical principle and then made more efficient. A greater "conservation" of human effort, Taylor argued, would maximize the output of a factory or business. All work could be organized more productively, and the results of labour shared so that the interests of owners and workers would converge.[20] Charlie Chaplin wonderfully satirized the assembly line and what it required of workers in his classic film *Modern Times*.

Productivity is the bedrock of contemporary theories of economic growth. Those economies that are productively efficient grow and create wealth for their members. In Canada, for example, we have been told repeatedly that we are less productive than our neighbour to the south, that we must increase our productivity if we are to continue to maintain our standard of living.[21] But what does productivity mean? The physiologists who studied human energy would have found the question easy to answer.

We can think about productivity in two different ways, although both rely on the same principles.[22] Productivity increases when a given, and useful, output — a bushel of wheat, a computer, a university degree — is achieved by lowering the inputs. If, for example, we could educate the same number of university students just as well with fewer faculty members by using distance-learning technology that is less expensive than a faculty salary, the university would become more productive. You may have noticed the critical words "just as well" that are built into the productivity calculation. Understanding what we mean by "just as well" and measuring quality is, of course, the hidden but critically important challenge.

Productivity also increases when the same number of inputs produces a larger number of useful outputs. A faculty that remains the same size at the same cost but provides the same quality of education to larger and larger numbers of students has improved its productivity. A hospital that, with the same budget, treats larger numbers of patients as effectively as it treated a smaller number has increased its productivity. Notice again the intrinsic relationship of effectiveness to productive efficiency — we cannot understand efficiency unless we first understand effectiveness. Productivity increases when people make better use of the resources they have, including their time, to increase the quantity of work they can accomplish while maintaining the quality.

The science of management examines how people can use the available resources, or different mixes of available resources, to increase the work they can accomplish. Time-and-motion studies, reorganization of workspaces, reallocation of responsibilities — all examine the use of available resources to identify ways of increasing productivity. The physiologists who began the study of human energy more than a century ago did much the same. They debated, for example, the role of diet and nutrition in enhancing labour productivity. Which diet, they asked, was appropriate for the optimal performance of the worker? German physiologists pointed to the lack of protein in the diet of workers and wondered whether the English workers' diet of meat and wheat-floured bread could account for their superior productivity. The controversy culminated in the famous "Brot versus Kartoffel"

debate in the 1870s and 1880s, when physiologists calculated that a diet of carbohydrates should consist of roughly 70 percent bread and 30 percent potatoes and vegetables. The heavier weighting of bread, they suspected, would increase worker productivity.[23] The modern management tradition is the intellectual inheritor of this early work.

The development of the concept of productivity is separate from but closely related to efficiency. We could, for example, become more productive by eating more expensive food. Productivity would grow, but efficiency would not necessarily increase. Productive efficiency is more demanding: it requires that the costs of the inputs — in this case, the diets of those who produce more — remain the same, even though the mix of inputs can change. Bread could cost no more than potatoes if efficiency were to be maintained. Or, in a more draconian world, productive efficiency requires that production remain constant but the cost of the diet be reduced. In Canada, for much of this past decade, we have been asking our health-care sector to reduce its diet while providing the same amount of care.

The analysis of productive efficiency depends on the capacity to quantify, measure, and compare the costs of the resources that are required to produce a given unit, and the capacity to measure and evaluate the quality as well as the quantity of what is produced. The task of measurement is demanding but manageable when markets set prices that act as surrogates for these complex measures. Prices are easily compared: we know the prices of a loaf of bread and a bushel of potatoes, and can easily compare their costs. The analysis of productive efficiency often misses many of the unintended consequences of both the processes of production and the goods and services that are produced. Nevertheless, in the production of private goods for the marketplace, this kind of evaluation is both feasible and revealing. When concepts of productive efficiency are applied to public goods — to health care, education, safe water, good government — the challenges, as we shall see, are formidable. How can we measure and compare the production of Plato's virtuous citizen or his just government? Reformers at the beginning of the past century struggled with exactly this question.

If concepts of efficiency could be applied to the human machine, the industrial machine, and the industrial worker, then they logically could be extended to government.[24] In the United States at the turn of the past century, reformers struggled with the corruption and inefficiency of local government. In education, city-hall politics controlled who was chosen as a school trustee, and money for school construction and teachers was the object of the pulling and hauling of political partisanship within municipal governments. Party politics — and "bossism" — controlled the agenda of education, municipal services, and all the other local public goods that urban dwellers needed. Reformers, appalled by the graft, argued that the inefficiencies, the failures of local government, were the result of partisanship and machine politics, of democracy as it was lived and practised. They used as their rallying cry a demand for efficient government. Lest we think that the current marketization of our language in public life is new, that the language of efficiency is recent, the use of market terminology in the public sector was present more than a hundred years ago.

In the name of efficiency, reformers demanded an independent, non-partisan, merit-based bureaucracy to run municipal services. Woodrow Wilson urged that a sharp line be drawn between politics and administration: although elected officials should make the important political decisions in a democratic society, professional administrators should manage the delivery of public goods. Bureaus of municipal research — some private and some quasi-public — were established in more than fifty cities in the United States. William Allen, who set up the New York Bureau of Municipal Research in 1907, complained, in horror, that "almost without exception, so-called reform governments have emphasized goodness rather than efficiency!"[25] We can only imagine what Plato would have thought about that complaint. Allen's research staff would stand at the curb, watching municipal employees fill potholes in the streets, and design ways to improve efficiency. Even more to the point, the bureau's staff — in a prescient argument — thought of efficiency as the essential prerequisite to accountability.[26] As we shall see, they missed the complexities of the terrain where efficiency meets accountability.

Democratic politics, the reformers argued, required not only responsiveness to social goals, but also their implementation through the most efficient methods —

bureaucracies based on merit and rational administration.[27] The reformers largely succeeded: professional,
merit-based bureaucracies began to grow during the New
Deal, and they reshaped the delivery of public goods in
the United States and elsewhere. Efficiency was invoked
to escape politics, to depoliticize the provision of basic
public goods. Rationality was joined to efficiency in a
merit-based bureaucracy. The public sector, in other
words, became the repository of rationality and efficiency,
insulated from the inherently corrupt, inefficient, and
irrational world of politics. Efficiency and rationality
were beyond politics, to be realized through the highest
possible standards of administration. It is this concept of
administration that developed and put in place many of
the programs of public goods that governments worldwide provide to their citizens today. The introduction of
formal budgeting processes and merit pay was the great
innovation in the delivery of public goods, the most
important change in the state until the creation of public
markets, the revolution that is now under way in the
post-industrial state.

The irony should not be lost on those of us who live at
the dawn of the twenty-first century, one hundred years
after the Weberian rational-legal experiment in efficient
government began. Max Weber, the great sociologist writing early in the past century, treated the state as distinct
from all other institutions, because its coercion was legitimate. In the rational-legal state, one of the three
ideal-types he developed, legitimacy functioned through
laws and rules, and through bureaucracy, whose central

purpose was to provide rational and efficient, top-down, rule-governed management.[28] The association of the word "bureaucracy" with rationality and efficiency sounds, as Lewis Carroll said in *Alice's Adventures in Wonderland*, curiouser and curiouser to our post-industrial ears.

Our conversation today has turned the other way. Contemporary reformers allege that the public sector, insulated and immune from the discipline of competitive markets, free from the pressures of productive efficiencies, is the repository of inefficiency and irrationality. The same bureaucracies of the public sector are now the obstacle to the efficient delivery of public goods, not the solution. The solution, today's reformers argue, lies not in politics and not in bureaucracies that are captured by special interests — or that pursue their own interests — but in markets that allow citizens freely to pursue their self-interest. The axis of efficiency rotates from its external objective standards and turns inward to the satisfaction of citizens as consumers.

Internal Satisfaction and Rational Choice

A market is a social system in which individuals pursue their own self-interest through exchange with others whenever these trades are mutually beneficial. Suppose that I like ice cream but have a dozen apples, and you have a pint of ice cream but prefer apples. We could trade, and we would both be happier. Apples may be better for me, but I really do prefer ice cream, and that is what matters. In a market, people pursue their self-interest, however they define it for themselves. The criterion becomes internal, rather than external. Rational individuals make efficient choices when they increase their welfare. The central idea of all market models is that voluntary exchange among people who can make rational choices is the best way to achieve efficiency.[29]

Surprisingly, it is among the Greek philosophers, who lived at a time when markets operated in the shadow of the state, that we find the early development of calculations of self-interest, worked out in ancient times with little reference to exchange or commercial values. The hedonic calculus of the Greeks was the early forerunner of the Benthamite calculation of happiness.

The utilitarians, writing in the eighteenth and nineteenth centuries, drew on the hedonic calculus to turn Plato on his head. They put interests, happiness, and welfare at the centre of politics — rather than, as Plato argued, placing virtue at the centre of welfare. Self-interest, the utilitarians insisted, is the primary value. Jeremy Bentham argued that pleasure and pain are the determinants of both natural and reasoned behaviour. People seek to maximize their pleasure and minimize their pain. It was a short step to substitute utility for pleasure and pain. As utilitarian arguments developed, they encompassed any goal that provides satisfaction. Efficiency turned inward and became silent about values, neutral about goals, but vocal about means. It became silent about values because what matters is what I value, not what is good for me. It became neutral about goals because what matters is whether I increase my satisfaction, whatever my purpose. It became vocal about means because all that can be evaluated is whether I made the efficient choice, given my values and my goals. With this turn in the conversation, we come to modern times.

Efficiency as the maximization of utility or satisfaction is quite different from the efficiency that is used to describe increased productivity. But the two are frequently confused in public conversation. Productive efficiency requires some external standard — how many pins per day does the factory worker produce? — while utilitarian arguments depend on internal standards — satisfaction, utility.[30] We may increase our productive efficiency but significantly reduce our utility. We may, for example, produce more energy by burning more coal at the same cost than we did a decade ago, but we significantly reduce our enjoyment of the countryside that is blanketed by smog. If enjoyment of the countryside matters more to us than the gain in productivity, then we have diminished our utility. An increase in productive efficiency would consequently be inefficient.[31] The concept of efficiency defined as the pursuit of self-interest is much broader than that of "productive efficiency," which economists use to explain economic growth. The two are not at all equivalent.

From this concept of maximizing our utility grew the contemporary concept of rational choice. The overarching assumption that governs much of the analysis of human behaviour today is that individuals have preferences and they generally make rational, efficient choices to maximize these preferences — neatly summarized as utility. How does it work? If I have to choose between two

hotels for my vacation, I will rank my preferences, compare the likely costs and benefits of each of the hotels, and
then rationally choose the one that is most likely to best
increase my satisfaction. Even if few of us actually make
our choices this way (and most of us don't), it is this picture of the rational decision-maker that is at the core of
market dynamics, and increasingly, of our explanations of
public choice as well.

Indeed, thinking about rationality in the modern age
has narrowed to thinking about rational choices, or efficiency. As the Nobel Prize–winning economist Amartya
Sen trenchantly observed, rational-choice models build
a picture of people as "rational fools," incapable of
differentiating among values, interests, emotions, and
commitments.[32] No one from Plato to Descartes would
recognize this portrait of rationality. To put it another
way, the writ of efficiency has expanded to subsume
rationality.

The concept of rational, efficient choice has migrated
from the individual to the consumer in the marketplace to
the leaders of states. Whether the subject is the prevention
of nuclear war or an outbreak of vicious ethnic violence,
scholars draw on the concept of rational, efficient choice
to explain the decisions leaders make.

For example, six months before the Cuban Missile
Crisis erupted in October 1962, as tension was escalating
between the United States and the then Soviet Union,
General Curtis LeMay came to see President Kennedy in
the Oval Office. The United States, he told the president,

had an 18:1 superiority in nuclear warheads. This was the moment, he insisted, to obliterate the Soviet nuclear force and, indeed, to delay for decades the emergence of the Soviet Union as a nuclear competitor to the United States. General LeMay urged the president to seize the first available opportunity to launch a nuclear attack against Soviet forces. President Kennedy thought for a moment, and then he asked LeMay what the cost to the United States would be: Would the Soviet Union be able to retaliate? General LeMay assured the president that "at the most, the United States would lose only three cities." The numbers were clear: the rational choice — obviously efficient — was to attack when the next crisis erupted. President Kennedy replied in the firmest possible voice, "Even one city is too much," and refused to meet with LeMay again. He rejected any suggestion of a nuclear attack, even when the costs to the Soviet Union would have been proportionately far greater.[33]

Those who choose to explain the president's decision with the language of efficiency would argue that Kennedy gave great weight to American lives in his utility calculus. That is the only way the numbers work, given the huge asymmetry in nuclear weapons and the high likelihood that the United States would have come out far better than the Soviet Union from any nuclear exchange. You and I might conclude that the president's values precluded the use of nuclear force. I suspect that, if we could ask him, Plato would be more comfortable with this explanation. The explanation of Kennedy's efficient, rational decision buries the values in the larger calculation. Our public conversation becomes largely instrumental — and diminished.

What happens in society when each individual maximizes his or her utility? Reasoning directly from the individual to the collective — not without great difficulty, as we shall see — Bentham put happiness as the unqualified end of politics.[34] The principle, Bentham argued, "states the greatest happiness of all those whose interest is in question, as being the right and proper, and only right and proper and universally desirable, end of human action: of human action in every situation, and in particular that of a functionary or set of functionaries exercising the powers of Government."[35] Government can be judged by its capacity to produce happiness, or the maximization of pleasure and the minimization of pain for the greatest number. The measure of good government, Bentham concluded, was whether "the tendency it has to augment the happiness of the community is greater than any which it has to diminish it."[36]

Bentham, unlike some of his successors who developed the thinking of Adam Smith, was troubled about the capacity of the free market to maximize the greatest happiness for the greatest number. Extreme inequality among citizens, he acknowledged, inhibits the maximization of happiness because the increase of pleasure derived by the rich from a given increase in income is far lower than that experienced by the poor. Bentham was making the now well-known argument of diminishing marginal utility: a decrease in the price of cooking oil — achieved, of course, through productive efficiency — will matter much more to a Cairean in one of the poorest neighbourhoods than it will to a wealthy merchant living in Giza. Bentham put his finger on a critical social problem in the concept of efficiency: collective efficiency is achieved only when it is no longer possible to increase the satisfaction of one person without decreasing the satisfaction of another.[37]

Bentham's shift from external to internal standards, and from the individual to the collective, is still at the core of much contemporary thinking about efficiency. An emphasis on individual satisfaction empowers the individual. The second — the movement from maximizing individual utility to maximizing collective utility — turns out to be very difficult, and fraught with paradox. A classic example of such a paradox is voting. Unless I get satisfaction from the act of voting itself, it makes little sense for me to expend the resources to go to the polling booth, since my vote is unlikely to influence the outcome of the election — unless I was living in Florida in November 2000. Nor does voting increase my productivity if I have to take time off work to go to the polls. The paradox is that if all voters made this same calculation of efficiency, no one would vote, and democratic elections would disappear. Individually efficient — and rational — decisions often produce collectively irrational outcomes. I may calculate accurately that enough Canadians who care about voting — who value democracy and the exercise of their vote — will go to the polls. I can stay home and be confident that democracy will survive in Canada. My calculation would be correct. I could free-ride.

You will notice that these paradoxes would disappear

if I valued the act of voting for its own sake. Remember that when it is used as an internal standard, efficiency is silent about values and neutral about goals. When the language of efficiency shapes the conversation, the gap between an individual's rational pursuit of self-interest and collectively efficient outcomes creates recurrent and serious problems in the delivery of public goods. Private benefits can create social costs — I stay at home and don't vote — and social benefits often require private sacrifices — I pay higher taxes so that my local lake can be cleaned up and restored. These "collective action" problems can be resolved — and sometimes simply managed — only through the exercise of public authority.

The utilitarians, when they made their arguments about universal self-interest, were making a political point as well as an economic argument. It may sound strange to our contemporary ears to say that the utilitarians were radicals, that many had an active political program of change. Axel van den Berg at McGill University puts it well:

> Today it is almost impossible to imagine — especially for those who see the world as divided between the poor masses and their corporate exploiters — that once upon a time the doctrine of the "free" market was profoundly *subversive*. But it was, and quite deliberately so. The ideal of a self-regulating market, in which people would be free to pursue their interests as they saw fit without interference from church or state, . . . was meant and understood as an eminently *emancipatory* doctrine.[38]

The concepts of universal self-interest and the maximization of utility, as Smith and Bentham developed them, were, and still are, profoundly radical. They were intended to subvert established political authority. A long line of thinkers — from Adam Smith and the classical political economists to contemporary critics of the state — saw the individual pursuit of self-interest as the most promising way to curb the power of monarchs, lords, and church in their pursuit of honour and glory.[39] The "free" market that resulted from the pursuit of self-interest was conceived, Albert Hirschman, the great political economist, observes, as the only reliable way "to restrain the arbitrary actions and excessive power plays of sovereigns."[40] Some — such as Adam Smith — saw little room for government at all, while utilitarians — such as Jeremy Bentham — in their drive for reform, attacked the traditional elitist, "unproductive" classes that controlled government. Here begin the faint murmurs of a refrain that would grow to cult status in our times: efficiency becomes the code word for an attack on government as a provider of public goods.

There is a second component to the political agenda of the utilitarians that also strikes an atonal chord in our contemporary ears. If all individuals had the capacity to pursue their self-interest, then all interests were inherently equal. As Stephen Holmes, a political historian, astutely observes, "Only a few have hereditary privileges, but everyone has interests. . . . To say that all individuals were motivated by self-interest was to universalize the status of the common man."[41] One interest had no inherent moral — or political — superiority over any other.

The utilitarian project is also empowering of the individual and profoundly optimistic about human capacity. Underlying the concept of the universal pursuit of self-interest is the argument that, given access to the information they need, individuals have the capacity to make rational or efficient choices, that we know best what is best for ourselves.[42] I know that ice cream is better for me at the end of a long day than an apple. This assumption of self-knowledge is, of course, a powerful argument for human liberty, individual responsibility, and human agency and choice. It is an argument for efficacy as well as efficiency.

Whatever the limitations of a concept of individuals as self-interested actors, however much it leaves out, it does generate a powerful sense of optimism and capacity. The empowerment of individuals to act on their own behalf and on behalf of their communities is among the most important requirements of a democratic society. We need a sense of optimism and self-confidence that we can indeed make the judgements and the choices that have to be made about public goods. As citizens, we must have a sense of efficacy.

Efficiency in the Market and the State: Public Markets

Our leaders, our commentators, our press argue passionately about whether the state or the market is the most efficient provider of our public goods — our roads, our water, our health care, our education. About private goods, of course, there is no longer any argument: in post-industrial society; the market reigns supreme and unchallenged. It is in the realm of public goods, the goods available to all, that the debate rages. Arguments that often seem to be local and even parochial — about local public education and home care and prescription drugs — are the tip of the iceberg of a much deeper, and profoundly important, debate about the appropriate roles of the state and the market in contemporary society. This debate, not surprisingly, is often couched in the language of efficiency. Again, not surprisingly, the language we choose to frame our arguments shapes the terms of the argument.

Very rarely do defenders of the state argue that it is efficient in providing public goods. They argue that it does so more equitably, more fairly, more justly than does the market. Some argue that the market cannot provide some public goods at all, and in these cases, the state is not the provider of choice but the only available provider. Here is a recent — and unusual — defence of the state as an efficient provider of public goods by an admirer of the market as an efficient provider of private goods:

> Far from serving as a drag on the economy, the state makes a huge contribution to the efficiency of the economy. It does so not only indirectly, by providing the background conditions needed for a flourishing market economy, but also directly . . . by providing goods and services that are not available in the private sector. The state lays just as many golden eggs as the market.[43]

The critics of the state do not buy this argument.
Adam Smith, Friedrich von Hayek, and in our own time,
Milton Friedman all argued passionately against the state
as the provider of public goods.[44] The state, they insisted,
gets in the way of individuals who, in the pursuit of their
own interest, would collectively pursue the common
good. The state, by distorting the market, creates massive
inefficiencies. Adam Smith delivered a stinging indict-
ment of the conceit of the state as a provider of public
goods:

> The man of system . . . is apt to be very wise in his own
> conceit; and is often so enamoured with the supposed
> beauty of his own ideal plan for government, that he can-
> not suffer the smallest deviation from any part of it. . . . He
> seems to imagine that he can arrange the different mem-
> bers of a great society with as much ease as the hand that
> arranges the different pieces upon the chess-board which
> have no other principles of motion besides that which the
> hand impresses upon them; but that, in the great chess-
> board of human society, every single piece has a principle
> of motion of its own, altogether different from that which
> the legislature might choose to impress upon it.[45]

Contemporary utilitarians — and others as well —
agree that when the state provides public goods, it creates
perverse, unintended consequences. Why? Because government leaders and officials have private interests of
their own, or are captured by others who use the state to
further their interests. "The idea of universal self-interest,

as it was used at the time of Adam Smith," Stephen
Holmes explains, "had a political rationale. It suggested
that citizens should distrust every expression of disinter-
estedness on the part of authorities."[46] Teachers' unions
capture bureaucrats and ministers who manage public
education, and those who manage universal health care
are captured by the interests of health-care providers. In
the process, the elusive and illusory common good suf-
fers. Indeed, the concept of the common good itself
becomes suspect. Much of this critique has been developed and expanded by scholars using theories of public
choice. They first demonstrate the inefficiencies of government, owing largely to the failure to get the
information it needs, but also, far more seriously, the per-
version of interests.[47]

Even without assuming malevolence, even if we sus-
pend disbelief and assume that the state is neutral, or
even benign, as early theorists of pluralism suggested,
critics still conclude that the costs of government management often exceed its benefits. Public management is
— the most damnable sin — inefficient. As Robert
Mundell, the Nobel Prize–winning economist, put it
recently, "Whatever you let government run, it runs
badly."[48]

If the state cannot provide — efficiently — the public
goods that citizens need and expect, then does the solution lie with markets? The history of markets suggests
otherwise; it tells of persistent inefficiency in providing
public goods. Even when we need public goods to
increase the efficiency of markets, Douglass North, an

historian of the global economy, argues, there is no individual incentive in the marketplace to supply public goods.[49] Rather, people, like our self-interested voter, tend to "free-ride" in the expectation that others will bear the cost. In modern society, it is states that have generally borne the cost of creating and supplying public goods.

It is not only self-interest that gets in the way of markets supplying public goods — it is markets themselves. Even the early proponents of markets recognized that a truly free market is an ideal construction that is rarely realized. "People of the same trade," Adam Smith wryly observed, "seldom meet together, even for merriment and diversion, but the conversation ends in a conspiracy against the public, or in some contrivance to raise prices."[50] Critics go further. They argue that imperfect competition, monopolies, price fixing, collusion, and cartels distort markets and enshrine inequalities, as well as producing inefficiencies, even in private markets. "Perfect" competition, just like the Weberian "rational-legal" state, is an illusion, an ideal that is not only unrealized, but unrealizable.[51]

The utilitarian project to limit — through the market — the arbitrary power of traditionally powerful groups that controlled the state paradoxically created new social inequalities. These inequalities might be tolerable in private markets in order to create still greater wealth, but they would be broadly unacceptable in markets for public goods embedded in societies that value equity, fairness, and justice. The earliest utilitarians — Bentham and his followers — anticipated the inequalities created by markets.

Governments responsible for the greatest happiness of the greatest number, Bentham argued, should provide abundance, security, and equity.[52] The free market efficiently promotes productive labour by encouraging the pursuit of self-interest, and the state, by guaranteeing the right to private property, provides security. However, Bentham argued, the extreme inequality among citizens that markets magnify inhibits the maximization of happiness. Government consequently has a role in reducing the extreme inequalities that diminish collective utility:

> I have never nor ever shall have, any horror . . . of the hand of government in economic matters. . . . The interference of government, as often as . . . the smallest balance on the side of advantage is the result, is an event I witness with altogether as much satisfaction as I should its forbearance, and with much more than I should its negligence.[53]

Bentham looked to democratic representation to check the private, "sinister" interests of elites that could capture government and to strict accountability in public bureaucracies. In joining efficiency and accountability at the hip, Bentham presciently prefigured much of the contemporary debate about the appropriate role of government as a provider of public goods.

The arguments that the champions of markets and the proponents of states each put forward to correct the structural inefficiencies created by the other are largely a dialogue of the deaf. Axel van den Berg brilliantly describes much of the contemporary debate as a debate among utopians who pay little attention to their respective "dys-utopias":

> Each side seems quite content to concentrate on unmasking the pretensions and hypocrisies of the other rather than examining the empirical validity of their own assumptions about their favoured solutions. Free-marketers continue to compare real, inefficient, parasitic, predatory, and corrupt governments with the textbook perfectly competitive market, whereas proponents of state interventionism keep comparing the rapacity and inequality of real markets with the perfectly democratic state.[54]

Large-scale organizations, van den Berg concludes, especially political structures, will almost naturally tend towards oligarchy just as markets will naturally tend towards oligopoly. Each — and both — will produce at times different and at times complementary inefficiencies.

Structural inefficiencies, although of different kinds, are, not surprisingly, the norm in both markets and states. The practice always differs from the ideal. When public rather than private goods are at stake, markets are even less likely to approximate the ideal of free and unfettered competition, and states are less likely to meet the standards idealized by Weber of rationality and efficiency. When we think about some of our most fundamental public goods — universal health care and public education — the critical question then becomes, What reduces the shared tendency to inefficiency and distortion? What combinations of state and market are most likely to mitigate the tendencies of the other? How can the one restrain the other, while capturing the advantages that each provides?

The contemporary answer in post-industrial society is to create public markets. What is a public market? Joining "market" with "public" seems like a contradiction in terms. It certainly is not a market that is set up in a public square, as one of my students suggested recently. A public market is created by governments: government provides public money and, either directly or through an arm's-length agency, invites providers to compete for contracts to supply a public good. For example, you rarely see government-owned bulldozers building highways. Governments invite private contractors to bid to build the road. Generally, the contractor who promises to build the road for the lowest cost wins the contract. This kind of process creates a public market where the purchaser — the state or its representative — is separated from the provider.

For some kinds of public goods — highways, coffee service in government buildings — establishing a public market is relatively straightforward. In education and health care, as we shall see, creating a public market and setting the rules for who can participate, and on what terms, is far more difficult. Any market, private or public, needs rules before it can begin to work; without well-developed laws of property, enforced by the state, no private market could function. We need only look at the difficult first few years in Russia after the collapse of the Soviet regime for a vivid example of the importance of the state to any market. In a public market, far more than any private market, the rules are the object of fierce political controversy.

Why create public markets? The state creates a public market in order to stimulate competition among the providers who supply the public goods. It is competition that supposedly is the prerequisite to efficiency, and public markets promise efficiency in the delivery of public goods. This is an ambitious and seductive promise, a promise that, if fulfilled, could transcend the centuries-long debate between the state and the market.

I want to explore whether public markets deliver what they promise. Do they provide efficiency in the delivery of public goods? And what happens to the state in public markets? Does the face it shows to its citizens change, almost beyond recognition? Even more to the point, I want to ask whether the language of efficiency is adequate to frame our conversation about the public goods that citizens need. I believe that it is not, and that it needs to be joined and matched by the language of accountability. Not without irony, public markets create the opportunity for a new agenda of public accountability. They also engage a broader discussion between proponents of a growing culture of choice that simultaneously joins and challenges the culture of rights.

II

EFFICIENCY AND ACCOUNTABILITY IN THE POST-INDUSTRIAL AGE

Late capitalism may prove unable to integrate the postmodern culture with its technological base. This is because the efficiency values of . . . [technology] are difficult to reconcile with a culture of narcissism. . . .

— John O'Neill[1]

Efficiency is a value. And whether we realize it or not, it is the central value in Canadian society.

— Joseph Heath[2]

THE RECENT EMERGENCE of efficiency as a cult is puzzling. Why now? Well into the past century, markets provided private goods, but the state — as the embodiment of rational, efficient administration — was still the provider of choice for public goods. It is only in the past quarter century, as post-industrial economies developed, that efficiency, coupled with markets, has come to dominate our conversation about public goods.

What explains our obsessive preoccupation with efficiency? In this chapter we will explore how, in the past
three decades, political, economic, and social forces
converged to elevate efficiency to a central value. Globalization has pushed markets and their language of
efficiency to the forefront of public consciousness. Even
more important, the transition to post-industrial society
and the emergence of knowledge as our most important
economic resource have enabled a shift in values from the
collective to the individual among citizens. It is post-
industrial society that has deepened public discourse
about efficiency and reshaped the face the state shows to
its citizens.

Talk about efficiency is only the beginning of our contemporary conversation. That language, as we will see in
this chapter, opens the doors to a much deeper discussion
about accountability, about choice, and about rights. Once
we have explored the currents that feed the stream of our
public conversation about efficiency, we can examine the
adequacy of efficiency as public language, and uncover
its intimate connections to the way we think and talk
about accountability. Our changing concepts of accountability will be, I suspect, one of the most important
battlegrounds of democratic debate and development,
and one of the lasting contributions of our current preoccupation with efficiency.

Accelerating Globalization

The globalization of markets and trade had intensified
long before the Cold War ended, but the public began to

pay attention to "globalization" only when the Berlin Wall fell and the threat of a large-scale nuclear confrontation between the two superpowers faded from public consciousness. Fifteen years ago, there was only a handful of books with the word "globalization" in the title. Today, there are thousands every year.

A decade ago, Francis Fukuyama could write a book with the revealing — and deeply misleading — title, *The End of History and the Last Man*.[3] Fukuyama expected that the collapse of the Soviet Union would end the era of great ideological conflict and that politics would be normalized. He was wrong: ideological conflicts continue, as they always will, but through different voices and agendas in post-industrial space. Globalization finds expression in a new language, new conceptions of borders and space, new kinds of networked organizations that work across state borders, new kinds of ideological controversies, and new kinds of conflict and violence.

Although globalization is currently a flashpoint of ideological controversy, protest, and violence, there is little agreement about what it is and what it means. Globalization can mean the integration of markets and the integration of production through large multinational corporations; it is these global markets and firms that enshrine the value of efficiency. This is how globalization is conventionally understood. It can also mean cultural hegemony, particularly the export of U.S. cultural products worldwide, along with American values and iconography. People in remote locations watch CNN news but also see the commercials and listen to the discussions of American politics and culture. Globalization also refers to the development of shared thought, language, and symbols among people who increasingly work wherever they want and live in no one place for very long. We usually think of scientific, technological, commercial, and financial elites as globalized minds, but members of humanitarian non-governmental organizations and human-rights organizations share this global sensibility, even though they give it very different meaning. The sense of home as place diminishes among these people, who increasingly think of themselves as global citizens, with global interests and values.

I think about globalization as the shrinking of distance through thickening networks of connections. It is the economic, technological, environmental, social, cultural, and political processes that work together first to connect and then to integrate the layers of societies. These linked processes, which are often mutually reinforcing, change established structures, languages, values, and institutions.

These processes of connection and integration are hardly new. The Roman Empire connected and integrated societies from Edinburgh to Jerusalem. Globalization has proceeded with fits and starts throughout history at an irregular pace and with uneven intensity, and it accelerated again in the second half of the past century. It began in the 1950s with the reduction of trade barriers through round after round of multilateral trade negotiations under the General Agreement on Tariffs and Trade (GATT). The lowering of trade barriers was followed by the elimination of restrictions on the flows of capital and the deregulation of financial markets. Globalization deepened further as direct foreign investment grew worldwide and multinational enterprises spread their chains of production. A new and powerful institution, the World Trade Organization (WTO), was created with unprecedented authority, through its capacity to regulate, to reach more deeply into domestic society than any of its predecessors.

More and more, national economies are being integrated into a single global marketplace through trade, finance, production, and a dense web of international treaties and institutions. Efficiency is the official watchword of global markets, and it is the governing orthodoxy of the thickening network of international institutions that seek to manage the global economy. Leaders of these newly powerful international institutions have enshrined market liberalism as official doctrine, and they promote efficiency in their programs and through their regulations. "Globalization of the mind," especially among commercial, financial, and technological elites, fuels the cult of efficiency.[4] Markets drive the global economy, while politics and law seek to regulate the markets they are chasing. It is no surprise that the language of efficiency, the watchword of markets, has become a global language.

The language of efficiency became part of public consciousness, surprisingly, before the latest round of globalization intensified, and even before the market liberalism of Margaret Thatcher and Ronald Reagan in the early 1980s. It did not come into public awareness in the way that we would expect. I think that we can credit the contemporary environmental movement for introducing efficiency into our public language. When Rachel Carson's groundbreaking book about pollution, *Silent Spring*, was published in 1962, public concern about the plundering of our natural environment exploded. Mounting evidence of pollution led naturally to discussions first of "waste," then of "conservation," and then of efficiency as a means of protecting and preserving our natural heritage. Public attention turned increasingly to "sustainable development," preventing waste, and the efficient use of environmental resources. Later, vivid examples of environmental damage — the meltdown of the nuclear reactor at Chernobyl in April 1986 and the growing hole in the ozone layer — gave environmental issues a central place on the public agenda. Solar heating, fuel-efficient automobiles, and recycling became part of the daily lives of many people. And all were justified in the language of efficiency.

Through the environmental movement, efficiency entered into public language as far more than a technical concept that is the preserve of specialized economists. Environmentalists made efficiency a moral imperative in the struggle to reverse a flawed conception of the relationship of the human species to nature. The human conceit that nature could be controlled was born of modernity and flourished in the machine age. In post-industrial society, waste is not only an economic issue, but a moral and — for some — theological issue that goes to the core of the conception of the human responsibility to nature. It was the environmentalists who enshrined efficiency as a virtue and waste as a public sin two decades before globalization rippled through public consciousness.

Market language also speaks of efficiency as a virtue, but in a very different, at times diametrically opposite, way from the language of environmentalists. It glorifies productive efficiency and, particularly in the post-industrial age, the efficient production of knowledge. In the past two hundred years, the most advanced economies have evolved from dependence on natural resources to the processing of these resources and the development of an industrial structure. In our age, knowledge has replaced other factors of production as the most significant commodity; the advanced economies now lead because of their capacity to innovate, to create, and to draw on and expand existing knowledge.

Unlike commodities that were important at earlier phases in economic history, knowledge is an infinitely renewable resource, only loosely related to geographical space.[5] We live in revolutionary times; today, unlike earlier periods in history, the more knowledge we use and create, the more we have. For the first time in history, we do not deplete our most important resource when we use it: the waste and conservation of knowledge are not concerns.

Knowledge is infinitely renewable and expandable, and it is also increasingly specialized and customized. We think very differently about "product" today than we have in the past. For example, at first it was those who grew tea and sold it abroad who reaped economic gain. Later, it was those who manufactured the teacup, mass-produced for a mass market, who profited even more. Consumers had little choice in what they bought once the industrial revolution gained force. But today, the standard model, made for mass consumption through mass production, is fast disappearing. What we produce today is tailored and individualized, customized and adjusted as we generate and export our knowledge. Knowledge products and services are targeted to niche markets, whether it is software design, biotechnology, or the customization of learning packages.

In the post-industrial, knowledge-based economy, we are less separated from our work than ever, for we work more and more in our minds. Everything is infinitely possible in the human mind, and we are moving into a world where what is internally possible is becoming externally conceivable. This expanding sense of possibility, as we shall see, fosters a sense of independence, autonomy, and a demand for choice among citizens. And as diversity, customization, and choice deepen in the private marketplace, they cannot help but spill over into demands for the same kinds of customization and choice in public goods.

It is not only the shape of private goods that is changing in the global knowledge-based economy, but the way they are delivered. Knowledge products and services increasingly move through networks and other horizontal forms of organization. The way we produce knowledge today is very different from the way pins were made in the factory Adam Smith visited. Here too, these new modes of delivery in the global marketplace cannot help but have an influence on the way public goods are delivered. New post-industrial forms of organization and delivery are challenging the traditional hierarchical command-and-control state that, for a century, delivered public goods in the industrial age.[6]

It is no surprise that ideological debate rages about the scope and consequences of contemporary globalization. Critics of globalization argue that it narrows the scope and autonomy of the state, that it constrains what states can do, and that it limits the capacity of governments to deliver the public goods that citizens have come to expect in the past half century. Today, the continuing economic and political pre-eminence of the state is no longer accepted conventional wisdom; some even predict an end to the era of the modern state.

This kind of argument does not stand up. The story is more complicated. Global markets and global politics are certainly deepening, but they do not constrain the state from fulfilling its social contract with its citizens. States still have real and significant capacity to provide public goods.

Those who argue that globalization weakens the state and limits its capacity to provide public goods can point to some convincing evidence. Global capital and firms are able to migrate to environments that offer the most attractive climate for investment and the greatest opportunity for profit, while the nation-state is fixed and immobile.

National financial markets are certainly weaker in comparison with global financial markets, and states, disciplined by global capital markets, have less freedom than they once had to use the traditional instruments of monetary and fiscal policy to stimulate economic growth and control recessions.[7]

As globalization has deepened, control, although not authority, has migrated beyond the state. It has moved to an ever-widening network of international and transnational institutions and law, some newly created and others newly strengthened. The World Trade Organization, through its capacity to regulate, penetrates far more deeply into domestic jurisdiction than did the GATT, its predecessor. Although there has been an explosion of international agreements, treaties, and tribunals in recent years, most international institutions remain heavily bureaucratic, thickly insulated from popular pressures.[8] But they are not insulated from protest. In response to the broadening writ of international institutions, groups of citizens are mobilizing in fragile global networks to try to hold these institutions accountable. Thousands came to Seattle for the Ministerial Conference of the World Trade Organization in November 1999, to Prague in September 2000 for the summit of the International Monetary Fund and the World Bank, to Quebec City in April 2001 for the Summit of the Americas, and to the G-8 summit in Genoa in July 2001 to demand greater transparency from international institutions that make decisions behind closed doors, decisions that have important consequences for far-flung local societies.

Power has also migrated to non-governmental organizations and transnational associations that work across and through state borders. In Africa, for example, it was not governments but Médecins sans Frontières (Doctors Without Borders), a transnational non-governmental organization, that led the global campaign to reduce the price of drugs to fight AIDS in poor societies. Multinational pharmaceutical companies, international institutions, and non-governmental organizations have joined with national governments to seek collaborative solutions. In South Africa, where the AIDS epidemic rages most fiercely, solutions to local health problems can no longer be national. South Africans live today in overlapping communities of fate, and they cannot look only to their government to provide a fundamental public good at a price they can afford.

There is a growing mismatch between an increasingly globalized private sector, a transnational voluntary sector, and a public sector that is fixed and continues to operate largely at the national level.[9] The public sector traditionally has been responsible for social entitlements, and for the reduction of inequality within nation-states. The Keynesian welfare state, constructed to insure its citizens against the risks of private domestic markets, now faces a much more formidable challenge from global markets and global institutions.

States and their economies certainly are tied more and more deeply to global markets and institutions. But what are the consequences? Here, the controversies begin. Some argue that globalization makes it much more

difficult for national governments to fulfil their traditional responsibilities to provide a social safety net and
basic public goods.[10] The state, they insist, is becoming
increasingly hollow, precisely because its borders no
longer correspond broadly to "national" economic, cultural, and social spaces.[11] State borders have become more
porous and fluid, and goods and services, ideas and culture, easily travel across these borders. So too do new
kinds of transnational organizations and shadowy networks of crime, terrorism, and violence.

The disconnect is clear: political boundaries continue
to remain largely fixed, while cultural and economic
spaces are changing, expanding, and reshaping.[12] In this
changing landscape, many believe a continuing retreat by
the state from providing social protection is both
inevitable and irreversible. The state may then become
one among many institutions bidding for the loyalty of its
members in a competitive marketplace of public and private spaces.[13] Critics of globalization conclude that a
retreat by the state will have disturbing consequences for
its capacity to provide public goods and for legitimate
and accountable governance.

This is far too pessimistic a view. Processes of globalization do pose formidable challenges to the state — and
to the citizen. But states still matter.[14] To begin with, markets, even global markets, need states and the legal
protections that they provide. Without the state, and the
legal framework of property rights that only states can
provide, markets could not function at all. Markets and
states are joined at the hip.

The state is indeed changing its shape in post-industrial societies, but not in the way critics of globalization expect. Surprisingly, post-industrial states are not reducing the proportion of the gross domestic budget they spend. The increased financial discipline imposed by globalization has not had the expected impact of reducing the size of government in post-industrial countries. Even more surprising, globalization has not led to the convergence of fiscal policies, nor has it stimulated the much-feared race to the bottom, where governments compete to reduce their rates of taxation and spending.[15] Indeed, the governments of post-industrial societies that trade the most have the largest budgets as a proportion of gross national product.[16] What this tells us is that the governments of the most open economies, those most heavily engaged in the global economy, have the largest capacity to provide public goods to their citizens. Contrary to conventional wisdom, globalization has not reduced the capacity of the state to invest in public goods.

Although the post-industrial state has not reduced its investment in public goods, it is changing the way that it provides public goods to its citizens. It is turning to markets and, at times, facilitating the creation of public markets for public goods. This change in the face that the state is showing to its citizens is the most important change since the creation of the merit bureaucracy and the Keynesian welfare state, and it can be explained only partially by the growth of global markets and global institutions.

We need to look beyond global markets to the *language* of globalization; this language has been far more important than markets themselves in changing the face of the state and the way it delivers public goods. Globalization comes with a language of efficiency and a widespread change in values among citizens of post-industrial societies.

The Changing Values of Citizens

While processes of globalization were deepening in the latter half of the twentieth century, the political values of publics were also changing significantly.[17] Values are the bedrock of political and social life; they are our conceptions of the good, of what is desirable, of how social and political life should be configured, and they inform our judgements about public issues. That values should have changed is not surprising: social and political institutions designed for the industrial era fit uneasily with post-industrial politics in the context of a global economy.[18]

Values have shifted from the collective to the individual. Among publics in post-industrial states, there is an increased emphasis on individual autonomy, and a shift from "solidarity towards self-affirmation."[19] Better educated and relatively secure from want, individuals in post-industrial societies generally place less emphasis on economic security and more on post-materialist concerns, such as the need for self-expression, freedom, fulfilment, and the quality of life.[20] Praise for the post-industrial economy and its values comes from an unexpected source, the Italian socialist Antonio Negri:

In the past, labour depended on capital to provide the factory and all the tools of production. Today, we have all the tools we need to work in our heads. This is the end of the distinction between production and life — life and work have become the same thing. But it is not life that has been reduced to work, like in a totalitarian society. Instead it is work that has identified itself with life. . . . Free men who one day or another might think in a different way, because the raw material of production is thought. . . . For politics, the big question today is how to organize life. . . . Our challenge is to invent new forms for organizing liberty in life and production.[21]

Politics is becoming a project concerned as much with quality of life as with microeconomics, as much with liberty as with equality.

Among unionized workers in Canada, the shift away from traditional values of solidarity towards personal self-satisfaction, autonomy, and quality of life is surprisingly strong.[22] Even in the segment of the population most likely to promote the values of solidarity, there is significant movement toward individualism. This value shift is especially pronounced in the younger generation, not only within unions but also among the general population, and it is consistent across post-industrial states. It is this shift, I think, that contributes to the growing culture of choice in Canada. Choice is increasingly spoken of as a right. Choice as a right joins — not always comfortably — the rights revolution.

"The rights revolution," observed Michael Ignatieff in his 2000 Massey Lectures, "took off in the 1960s in all the industrialized countries, and it is still running its course."[23] The rights agenda, so prominent now in our public conversation, drew strength from the radical individualism of the post-industrial world, where citizens in the fortunate part of the globe struggle with the dilemmas of affluence rather than the challenges of necessity and survival. The culture of rights — embedded as civil rights and charter rights within many democratic societies — has broadened and deepened.

Rights talk has spilled over national borders into global politics and institutions. The Universal Declaration of Human Rights was proclaimed by the United Nations in 1948 in the wake of the terrible evils perpetrated by Nazi Germany. It was the first in a series of charters and international laws that gave individual rights precedence over state sovereignty when the state perpetrated evil. The public discussion of human rights, of rights that derive simply from being human, deepened during the Cold War as a tool in the broader critique of the Soviet Union. However, human rights as a concept quickly resonated beyond that particular political agenda.

"Human rights are the rights men and women have," Ignatieff argues, "when all else fails them."[24] The global rights revolution has led to the creation of special military tribunals to investigate war crimes committed in Yugoslavia and Rwanda, and to a new international criminal court. It has led to the prosecution of political leaders outside their own jurisdiction for crimes committed while they were in power. Political office no longer provides protection for crimes against humanity and genocide. The legal charges against Augusto Pinochet of Chile and Slobodan Milosevic of Yugoslavia for orders they issued while they were president testify to the broadening and deepening of the culture of human rights. The United Nations now has a commissioner for human rights, and non-governmental organizations such as Amnesty International and Human Rights Watch monitor the observance and violation of human rights around the world.

The universality, meaning, and observance of human rights are hotly contested not only by those who oppose, but also by those who defend, the global human-rights agenda. Yet during the past quarter century, the concept of individual human rights that trump the sovereignty of the state has become an accepted part of political rhetoric and public conversation. As with globalization, the growing importance of individual human rights does not leave the state untouched.

In a closely interconnected world, it has been but a short step to project these rights from those who enjoy them to those who don't. Respect for individual rights, the product of the politics of affluence in secure democracies, has become the prescribed solution to poverty and famine. "Individual agency," writes Amartya Sen, "is, ultimately, central to addressing these deprivations. . . . Expansion of freedom is viewed . . . both as the primary end and as the principal means of development. Development consists of the removal of various types of unfreedoms that leave people with little choice and little

opportunity of exercising their reasoned agency."[25] Freedom and human agency have become the solution for the
poor as well as the preoccupation of the affluent.

This shift to post-materialist values and a culture of
radical individualism among the affluent does not map
neatly onto the privatization of public life. Contrary to
what we might think, citizens are becoming more, not
less, interested in their government's role in providing
public goods and in political participation. But what we
expect and how we are engaging politically is changing.
Despite the increased importance of individual autonomy
and self-affirmation, citizens in Canada, as elsewhere in
the post-industrial world, continue to look to government
to assure the basic public goods that enhance the quality
of our lives. We also want government to provide better-
quality public goods more efficiently. But we are deeply
ambivalent about the role of the state: surveys tell us that
half of Canadians feel their government is trying to do too
much and should cut back.[26] We want government both to
do less and to do better.

In the past five years, there has been a profound
change in the priorities and public agenda of Canadians.
Until the mid-1990s, so few Canadians cited social issues
as the most important problem facing the country that
these issues did not even appear in the *Maclean's* annual
survey of the concerns of the Canadian public. In 1996,
social issues became the most important concern of
11 percent of the population; today, that number has
grown to almost 50 percent, as the most important social
issues — health care and education — eclipse any other

category by a ratio of more than 4:1.[27] More and more of what we call "quality of life" issues are at the centre of the public agenda.

The nature and purposes of public participation are also changing. Engagement in conventional politics is flat or declining; fewer people are participating actively in conventional politics than ever before. Fewer are turning out to vote and even fewer are loyal to political parties. However, more people are becoming involved in unconventional forms of political action.[28] There is a greater willingness by young people to participate in boycotts, demonstrations, and new social movements that challenge authority and established institutions. We need only look at the number of young Canadians who went to Quebec City for the Summit of the Americas in April 2001 for tangible evidence of the changing political values of some of our citizenry.

Why this willingness, especially among younger people, to engage in political activities that challenge established institutions? One reason is that citizens are generally dissatisfied with the ways their institutions work. Confidence in governmental institutions has fallen far more dramatically than, for example, confidence in large corporations.[29] Within unions, there is a parallel trend: members, especially younger members, are increasingly sceptical of the effectiveness of their national leaderships.[30] These trends are mirrored in other post-industrial states.[31] It is not surprising that a better-educated and more economically secure citizenry is less deferential to established authority structures and demands for itself both accountability and voice.

The political agenda is changing as well, at home and abroad. In Canada, as economic development has provided relative security for most of the population, support for policies that redistribute income and provide social benefits has fallen. This shift is most pronounced in societies that have the most advanced social legislation and the highest levels of income equality. In Denmark, for example, where progressive taxation is high and social supports extensive, support among the public for redistribution is the lowest in the European Union. In Greece, the poorest member of the EU, support for reducing income inequality is highest.[32] In Canada, where income inequality is less than that of its neighbour to the south, support for redistribution is falling as well.

The public does care — and cares deeply — about fundamental public goods such as health, education, and the environment, but it is also deeply dissatisfied with and distrustful of the institutions that are the traditional suppliers of these public goods. The younger, more educated citizenry feels capable of challenging established practices and developing alternatives, both at home and in the global marketplace and society. The watchwords are efficiency, accountability, and responsiveness — and increasingly, autonomy and choice.

The shape and interests of government are also changing. The new agenda of government is also accountability — as well as efficiency — but the thinking in government about accountability and efficiency differs in important ways from that of the public. The way these two agendas connect, and whether citizens and states come to consensus on the meaning of efficiency and accountability, will shape the politics — and the delivery of public goods — of the next quarter century.

The New Shape of the State: After the Factory

Governments are changing the ways they provide public goods to their citizens. As networks and horizontal production arrangements in the new knowledge-based economies have displaced the factory and the assembly line, the industrial model of the state, with its command-and-control bureaucracies, fits more and more uneasily into the landscape. The "factory" model of the state sits uncomfortably within organizations that emphasize learning, and among citizens who increasingly emphasize autonomy and choice. As the centrally controlled and hierarchically managed assembly line loses its prominence, states, in the argot of our times, are changing the way they "do business."

The traditional bureaucracy is organized as a hierarchy, adheres to rules and procedures, and pays attention to the prevention of waste. The new "post-bureaucratic" organization pays attention to quality and value, demand rather than supply, agreement on norms, and consensus on shared problems at the lowest possible levels within the organization.[33] The successful firm in the private sector provides the model for the organization of the state: self-reinforcing learning backed by accessible research, and the movement of decision making down to the lowest level, where people confront the full range of issues and dilemmas.[34] States are changing, slowly to be sure, from a command-and-control hierarchy to "learning" organizations, in partnership with others. Adjusting to the way firms are reorganizing and citizens think, states are getting "out of the business" of directly providing public goods. Less and less often do states deliver public goods directly through programs they manage and run.

The radical innovation of our time is the turn by the state to markets, public as well as private, to deliver public goods. Post-industrial states continue to finance public goods, but they have stepped back from directly delivering these goods to their citizens. Some are quite deliberately stimulating the creation of public markets, where providers of public goods compete directly for public money. The post-industrial state is increasingly a partner and contractor, working jointly with other institutions — private as well as public — to set the terms on which others deliver public goods. The state contracts out the work that it expects can be done more efficiently by others, whether that work is maintaining military bases, providing policing, delivering development assistance, supplying military training, managing prisons, running schools, providing security at airports, or delivering health care. The hope and the promise is that through the logic of markets, competition will increase efficiency. This change in the way the state works — through markets rather than as a manager and operator — is the most significant change since the development of the rational, efficient, bureaucratic state a century ago.[35]

The new role of the state as partner and contractor of

public goods brings with it new responsibilities. States set the terms of the contract, finance the services, and regulate the delivery of public goods. As regulators, they set standards for the quality of the public goods that they are buying, audit the efficiency with which public goods and services are delivered, and monitor the quality of the public goods that are provided. To accomplish these tasks, governments need to increase dramatically the information they have about quality: they need to learn in new ways about new issues. This creation of public markets through the split between purchaser and provider is changing the face government shows to its citizens.

With its new role and new responsibilities, the state matters to its citizens just as much if not more than before. The state may be less visible, but it is present. It remains the guardian of the quality of public goods, the "voice" of the public, and the standard-bearer of the public interest.[36]

The Language of Efficiency: Is It Adequate?

The concept of efficiency has had widely different meanings in different historical periods. It has often been used in explicit pursuit of political purposes: a technical discussion of efficiency and public goods — allegedly the concern of professional economists — is almost always embedded in a larger political agenda. Whether it was the pursuit of virtue in ancient times, or the creation of merit-based administration at the turn of the past century, or a frontal attack on the bureaucratic state and a turn to markets, as it frequently is today, efficiency has served as a rallying cry for larger political purposes. The allegedly technical concept of efficiency has been politically charged in every age. Our age is no exception.

But a terrible confusion between means and ends bedevils our contemporary public conversation about efficiency. Not so, argues economist Joseph Heath in his recent book on the efficient society. "Efficiency is a value. And whether we realize it or not, it is the central value in Canadian society. It has largely displaced religion, ethnicity, and language as a source of public loyalty." Efficiency is a value, he continues, because it is a criterion that we use to decide what is good and bad, what to choose, and because it tells us how we should do things.[37]

Heath's celebration of efficiency as a central value is misplaced. When means are disconnected from ends, the call for efficiency becomes a cult. Efficiency does not tell us where to go, a wise observer of politics once commented, only that we should arrive there with the least possible effort.[38] Efficiency is about how we should allocate our resources to achieve our goals, not what our goals should be. What our goals are, and how much we value them, is properly outside the language of efficiency. Indeed, contemporary utilitarians argue, one of the alleged strengths of using preferences as the basis of choice is that no value judgements are made about goals. The standards are internal to the chooser, and as we saw in chapter 1, efficiency is neutral about goals and silent about values.

We are not efficient for efficiency's sake.[39] Much of what we value, as the political analyst Edward Luttwak notes, lies outside the market — love, our community, comfortable old shoes. Efficiency has no inherent value. More than one-third of the population of Canada identifies maintaining our health-care system as the top public priority, and half the population is willing to consider moderate user fees or a private system alongside medicare. "But make no mistake," the pollster Allan Gregg argues, "it is our health standards that the population values and not user fees or private medicine. The problem to date has been that political leaders have been unable to convince the electorate that they share Canadians' understandings of what are ends and what are means."[40] Gregg is exactly right. This confusion between means and ends, between instruments and values, badly confounds our public conversation.

We begin with the assumption that in the delivery of public goods, efficiency *is* important as a means to achieve public ends. It *is* important to use efficient — or cost-effective — means to provide valued public goods so that public funds, which are never infinite and almost never adequate, can stretch to meet as effectively as possible the largest number of public needs. Embedded in the concept of productive efficiency is an assessment of quality and effectiveness, as well as quantity. Efficiency can mean productive efficiency, or cost-effectiveness, when either the maximum amount of a public good is produced from a given set of resources, or a given public good is produced with fewer resources.[41] Either way, the best possible use is made of available resources to achieve public ends.

The trade-off between efficiency and effectiveness, a

trade-off that we hear so much about in our public conversation, is blatantly nonsensical. Effectiveness is built
into any concept of efficiency. Before we can determine
whether we are efficient at providing universal health
care in Canada, we first need to establish whether
the health care that is being provided is effective. Is our
health-care system effective at health promotion and prevention of illness? Is it effective at assuring access? Is it
effective at pioneering surgical techniques?

We need to ask the same kinds of questions about
public education. Are our public schools effective? We
can't answer this question until we understand the purposes of education. Effective at what? At producing
literate students? At producing critical thinkers? At producing engaged young citizens? Would we want a system
of public education where the majority of our high-school
students know nothing of Canadian history or values but
excel at science and mathematics? What, in short, are the
goals of education and health care in Canada? Without a
discussion about the goals, and the values that inform
these goals, we cannot even begin to talk about efficiency.

We need answers to these questions about effectiveness *before* we can begin to do the calculation about
whether resources are being used efficiently in public
education. Judgements about effectiveness — extraordinarily difficult to make and always subject to political
contestation and debate — must logically precede any
calculation of the efficiency of means. It is no accident that
efficiency is often used to mean cost-effectiveness: it
relates cost to effectiveness. To think about efficiency, we

need to know *what* we want to accomplish and how important it is.

Even when efficiency is restricted properly to means, it is often used incorrectly in public discussion. Particularly in an age of fiscal austerity, efficiency is at times twisted by political leaders to mean cost-cutting or cost-containment. The error should be obvious: neither cost-cutting nor cost-containment is inherently efficient if the quality or the quantity of the public goods governments provide is reduced more than the costs. Distorting efficiency this way often masks a distrust of government as the custodian of the public interest and a political preference for markets as the providers of public as well as private goods. That is much of what we have heard lately in Canada, for example, in the testimony over the safety of our water.

If my logic is persuasive, then it should be clear that in the discussion of public goods, efficiency is an intensely political concept. Judgements about the effectiveness of public goods are inevitably laced with political claims, but without these judgements, no calculation of cost-effectiveness can be made. And these political judgements become more complex as we dig down into the calculus of efficiency. Technical language should not obscure the fundamentally political character of calculations of efficiency in public goods.

Efficiency also includes the allocation of resources to achieve public ends. Allocative efficiency exists when resources are distributed so that they are used in the best possible way.[42] How well are resources being used to accomplish the public purpose? Are resources going where they should? In Canada, are we distributing resources across the health-care system in the most efficient way? Is it efficient to insure acute care and leave very limited resources for home care as the population ages? Is it efficient to insure physicians' services but provide no public insurance for the services of physiotherapists outside of hospitals?

We also need to ask, Efficient for whom? Our public conversation frequently focuses, for example, on the artificial trade-off between efficiency and equity. We are told — wrongly — that we must choose between greater efficiency as an end and greater equity, also as an end. In his well-known book *Equality and Efficiency: The Big Trade-Off*, Arthur Okun argues that the competition in the American economy that creates efficiency also creates large inequalities.[43] But this is a badly misstated presentation of the problem when it comes to public goods. Properly stated, equity is the end and efficiency is the means. Very few citizens, I suspect, would want to spend public monies inefficiently on programs to promote equity.

There are four possible equations that we can imagine. We can be *inefficient at being inequitable*; this is a fair representation of health-care delivery in the United States. We can be *inefficient at being equitable*; this is a somewhat unfair representation of some of our human-resources programs in Canada. We can be *efficient at being inequitable*; this is a fair representation of the aspirations of the worst totalitarian governments in the past century. Finally, we can be *efficient at being equitable* — the

as-yet-unrealized utopian goal of all democratic governments that provide public goods.

The challenge of efficiency is not an easy one for public institutions to meet. In private markets, efficiency
increases through competition. Competition is the
dynamic that forces a constant, at times unrelenting,
increase in individual effort — a race to the top. Competitive markets discipline inefficient suppliers by providing
rapid feedback; buyers constantly seek more efficient
suppliers. This kind of competitive dynamic is not a
characteristic of the hierarchically organized command-
and-control bureaucracies that are the foundation of the
industrial state.

In practice, markets for private goods are often far
from competitive. Public markets, with a single payer —
the state — or with only a few powerful suppliers, are
never likely even to approximate the ideal of competition.
Public markets created to enhance competition can at best
only faintly echo the utopia of a genuinely free and open
market. The gap between the ideal of a free market and
the reality makes the concept of efficiency even more
problematic in public space than it is for private goods.

Careful conversation about efficiency — when it asks
the questions *efficient at what, how well,* and *for whom,*
when it moves beyond cult to engage in talk about public
purpose, helps to ask hard questions about public goods.
This kind of discussion requires admittedly difficult and
politicized judgements about quality, effectiveness, and
allocation of resources. Critics of government delivery
are right when they insist that we cannot afford to waste

scarce public funds through inefficiency, and critics of markets are right when they insist that a perfectly free market rarely exists for private goods, much less for public goods. The language of efficiency — when it is used appropriately as a calculus of the relative cost and distribution of resources to provide effective public goods — is a good beginning. It opens a conversation about what public goods are provided, how effectively they are provided, and to whom they are provided. Our post-industrial language of efficiency lets us ask some important political questions about public goods. This may be among its most important contributions.

Efficiency and Accountability

Even when the language of efficiency is used carefully, that language alone is not enough. Unilingualism will not do, as Jeremy Bentham argued. Efficiency in the provision of public goods needs to be joined by a conversation about accountability. States are facing newly intensified demands for accountability from their citizens. And it seems likely that these demands will grow as states turn to markets to provide public goods. Accountability is about evaluating performance, meeting legitimate standards, fulfilling legitimate commitments, and holding responsible those who fail to meet the standards. The right to judge government performance flows naturally from the role of citizen, as does the right to sanction those who fail to meet the standards.

Judging the performance of governments occurs through widely accepted — even if unsatisfactory —

political and legal processes. Holding to account private or public suppliers of public goods who are contracted by government is more challenging. The relationship is triangular rather than bilateral, with at times indirect and unclear lines of authority among citizens, those who provide public goods, and the state. Citizens rightly expect direct accountability from those who supply their most important public goods, but providers of public goods are formally accountable to those who purchase their services — the government — rather than directly to the public. The threads of accountability become even more tangled; the standards governments exact are not necessarily synonymous with the standards of citizens. In the cost-effectiveness equation, governments tend to pay more attention to cost than to effectiveness. And once a contract between the government (as purchaser) and a provider is in force, it becomes difficult, if not impossible, for citizens to end the contract early or to sanction the provider directly. To be fair, much the same can be said for the mandate we give governments in democratic systems. We elect governments for four to five years and cannot end their term early if they fail to meet our standards.

There are generic differences in the way citizens within democratic states and consumers in the private marketplace judge performance and sanction those who fail to meet standards. How each judges, and what is being judged, differs. In private markets, firms owe accountability first to their shareholders, who take precedence over consumers. As private consumers, if we are dissatisfied with the product or the service, we can only take our business elsewhere. The ability of a consumer to exercise accountability rests almost entirely on our capacity to "vote with our feet," on our capacity to exit. For some kinds of public goods, citizens can indeed exit the public system when they are dissatisfied with the quality it offers. They can send their children to private schools or go abroad for medical care, but often it is only a small proportion who can afford these private alternatives.[44]

What private consumers judge is also different. Within the constraints created by the regulations that govern the claims that producers can make, consumers have limited rights to information about the effectiveness of a good or a service. They are largely dependent on their own judgement of the quality and effectiveness of what they buy. Citizens, as consumers of public goods in a democratic state, are in a very different position. Government is accountable first and foremost to its citizens. And we have the right to know about the quality and effectiveness of public goods. The right of consumers to judge performance is embedded in private life and exercised through markets, but citizens' rights are constitutive of public life. The right to know about and judge performance, the right to responsiveness from those we have judged inadequate, and the right to sanction are fundamental attributes of citizenship in a mature liberal democracy.

Accountability to the public by those who provide public goods should not be a revolutionary concept. It is the foundation of all democratic theory. Yet this principle has generally been honoured far more in the breach than in the observance when it comes to those who directly provide public goods. Our educators, our schools, our universities, our hospitals, our physicians, our health-care providers — all are accountable to the public they serve. To hold them accountable, agreed standards must logically precede any evaluation and judgement of performance. The generic concept of "quality" — quality education, quality health care — is often invoked as a mantra, but it is given little meaning. Quality first has to be translated into standards of effectiveness and then used to evaluate public goods. But developing appropriate standards of effectiveness is neither easily done nor politically neutral. And what we choose to consider effective does matter. It matters because the standards used to measure effectiveness feed back and reshape not just what public goods are delivered, but how they are delivered.

Who chooses the standards of effectiveness? Do these standards reflect the preferences of citizens, of those who use the system, of professionals who provide the public goods, of experts who manage the system, or of governments that contract for the services? These are difficult issues, but they go to the heart of the exercise of accountability. Standards of effectiveness are politically contested, yet there is no alternative but to develop these criteria if we hope to hold public institutions and political leaders accountable.

Citizens in affluent democratic societies, who have had every opportunity, have generally failed to exercise their right to hold accountable those who provide basic public goods. In the next two chapters, I want to raise some questions that we might ask of our education and health-care providers, and of our political leaders responsible for the education and health care systems: *At what* are you efficient? *For whom* are you efficient? *For what* are you accountable? *How* are you accountable? And *to whom* are you accountable? If we as citizens cannot imagine how we can hold our local public school accountable — and for what — or how we can hold our neighbourhood clinic or the hospital down the street accountable — and for what — how can we begin to think seriously about holding our more distant and impersonal governments accountable? And if we cannot imagine how we hold our public institutions accountable, how can we expect responsiveness?

It is not only citizens that are changing, but also the face of the state. The new role of the state as contractor, regulator, and partner should make it both easier and more difficult for states to meet at least some of these demands for accountability. The state as contractor and regulator now has no choice when it enters into contracts but to specify, in advance and with some precision, exactly what kinds of services are expected and what kinds of standards must be met. This is the hard part, for governments often do not have this kind of comprehensive information before the fact. They must also collect information about the quality of the public goods and the efficiency with which they are delivered. The tragic results of the failure to collect information and monitor the performance of those who managed the water system in Walkerton, Ontario, and airport security across North

America provide eloquent warning.

We have arrived at a signal moment in history, when the demands of states and citizens seem to converge, at least in part, although for very different reasons. When the state was the sole deliverer of public goods, it had every incentive as a monopolist to conceal rather than reveal. The new post-industrial state needs transparency among providers, assurances of quality, and evaluations of the effectiveness of the public goods that are delivered. So do citizens.

The agendas of the contractor state and the public also diverge. As the state contracts out responsibilities for the delivery of public goods, many institutions — legislatures, committees — lose their capacity to monitor, investigate, and steer programs. And inevitably, private contractors will try to limit the amount and kind of information they provide — in the name of efficiency![45]

These new responsibilities of the state are likely to cause deep unease inside and outside governments. Accountability requires transparency, standards, open evaluation, a capacity to learn quickly and to correct deficiencies when they become apparent. Transparency is not typical, however, of hierarchical organizations that habitually respond to direction from the top, are acculturated to secrecy rather than openness, and in their capacities as custodians of the public interest, are deliberate and conservative rather than nimble in their ability to adapt. Contracting services can further reduce the flexibility of governments if the contracts are long term. These attributes fit poorly with the deepening public scepticism of governmental stewardship and the accelerating demands that governments be more accountable to the public.

Greater accountability is also likely to cause unease among the broader public. Governments will require newer and far more extensive information about performance than they have in the past. In health care and education, they will need access to information and evidence that many citizens consider private. It is in this sense that governments will be more, not less, present and more, not less, invasive. It is no coincidence that the government of Ontario recently announced that the provincial auditor general will have access to the accounts of institutions in the broader public sector — universities, hospitals, and the other "partners" that it finances. It is, after all, "our money" that is being spent, the auditor general remarked. As accountability deepens, fundamental questions about the privacy of citizens and the control and reach of governments will become increasingly important on the public agenda.

Governments will also inevitably become more coercive. They will become — to a greater or lesser extent — the "accountability police" of providers of public goods. To be accountable is to be held responsible for performance according to recognized and agreed-upon standards. If accountability is to have any meaning, standards must be explicit, and those who fail repeatedly to meet them must be helped to improve or, as a last resort, sanctioned. If providers are systematically inefficient at achieving their goals, then in the language of our times, they must be "put out of business."

The new state will be leading the discussion of accountability. If we are to avoid the inevitable excesses of an "accountability police," if we do not want to leave the determination of the terms and meaning of accountability exclusively to the state, citizens must join with experts and professionals in public discussion of the shape and substance of the standards that will be at the heart of the exercise of accountability. Determining what kind of test to give students in the third grade and whether the results are appropriate to judge the effectiveness of public education may seem either a trivial or a technical discussion; it is not. It is a microcosm of the larger conversation about the accountability of public institutions in a democratic society.

The critical question then becomes, Who defines the standards? Is accountability to be imposed or negotiated through a deliberative political process that gives voice to all the stakeholders in the new, far more complicated network of accountability? And do we have the capacity to negotiate accountability? Much of the democratic debate of the next decade will turn on whether accountability is imposed or negotiated. It is the next battleground for democratic theorists and practitioners.

The Culture of Choice and the Culture of Rights

Efficiency and accountability are embedded in the larger context of the rights revolution, and in a culture of choice that is growing as the post-industrial age deepens. The rights revolution, Michael Ignatieff explains, has been about both "enhancing our right to be equal and protecting our right to be different."[46] Canadians, like many others around the world, believe more and more that health care and education are rights. We have a right to health — *Health for All* is the title of a report issued by the World Health Organization — as well as a right to basic public education.

But we also claim the right to be different and particular — to choose the kind of education we want for our children, and even to choose our physician. By exercising the right to choose our schools and our doctors, we can at times compromise the rights of others. The right to choose a particular school may make the schools that are available to others less effective, and the right to choose our doctors may make medical care less cost-effective. Citizens value their right to public goods, but increasingly they also value their right to choose the kinds of public goods they want. These values may not always live well together.

The culture of choice, part of the larger tapestry of radical individualism, is nourished by the sense that government is insufficiently responsive, and that we as citizens are quite capable of making sound judgements on public issues. The culture of choice is growing as part of the rights revolution, but the two are not always compatible. This is a tension that is built into the post-industrial age as structures become less hierarchical and citizens become less deferential. It sets the context as governments struggle to find more efficient ways to provide public goods and as providers struggle to become more accountable. It is to this tension that we turn in the next chapter.

III

EFFICIENCY AND CHOICE: PUBLIC EDUCATION AND HEALTH CARE

If you want to start a good argument anywhere in Ontario, just utter the words "school choice." Then duck.

— Margaret Wente[1]

Conservatives will have to show that they — better than anyone else can match the service standards of global capitalism in providing the public goods that governments exist to provide.

— William Thorsell[2]

PUBLIC GOODS, as we have thought about them, are those goods that are not easily divisible. Nor can citizens be easily excluded from their benefits. Safe streets in the cities in which we live cannot be divided among the residents and are available to everyone to enjoy. To stimulate more efficient delivery of public goods, states in the post-industrial age are creating public markets. What are these public markets and how do they work? What do they promise and what do they deliver?

Public markets are created when the state moves from directly providing social protection and invites others — public institutions, private and not-for-profit organizations — to compete for government funds to supply a public good. The logic of a "public market" is clear: when the supplier (the provider of public goods) is separated from the buyer (the state or its representative), providers will compete to supply public goods and efficiency will increase. Competition is the magic that promises efficiency.

Listening to the conversation in our society about public markets is enlightening. The discussion about two of our most important public goods — public education and health care — tells us a great deal, both because these two public goods meet such important individual needs and because they reflect how we see ourselves, as citizens and as a society. As we listen, we can peel away the layers of the conversation to discover if public markets deliver what they promise. Are they efficient? If so, at what? At improving the quality of education and care? At providing access to education and health-care services? And, how is the term efficiency being used in our public conversation? Is the conversation really about efficiency at all, or is it a surrogate for other conversations about other values, conversations that we are not having? When we listen, what we find is surprising: public markets do not fulfil their promise of greater efficiency, but they do deliver the unexpected.

To listen to this conversation, I want to tune in to the talk about two among many different kinds of public markets. Both are, of course, publicly financed. The first allows public funding to follow the choices that citizens make as they "shop" for public goods, supplied by providers that work outside a framework of universal access. Radically new proposals for vouchers in education and medical savings accounts in health care are of this kind. So too, in a less direct way, are established two-tier medical systems. Competition for funding that follows citizens, the argument goes, will provide better public goods more efficiently, as inefficient providers are naturally forced out of the market.

A second kind of public market is more genuinely public. It requires public funding to flow only to public institutions or to private providers that work within a set of rules that provides universal access. This kind of market has more restrictive rules governed by an explicit normative framework — a commitment to universal access and equity. In this sense, it is a new breed of market. Charter schools in education and public markets for health care in Britain use market logic within the framework of a commitment to universal access and equity. Public funding is common to both kinds of markets, but their rules are very different, with different consequences for how resources are allocated and public goods are delivered, and for society as a whole.

The role of citizens in these markets is politically controversial. In mature liberal democracies, we generally describe ourselves as citizens with rights, not as "consumers" of public goods. When we go to the emergency room of our local hospital with an urgent complaint, we go first as patients and then as citizens, with the expectation that we have a right to health care as a public good. Many make this argument of the primacy of citizenship in the often bitter debate with the unwavering defenders of markets in post-industrial societies. This argument captures an important constitutive element that distinguishes public from private life, but it is also misleading.

As citizens, we are consumers of public goods. Indeed, it is precisely as citizens that we are entitled to be consumers of public goods. Every time we send our children off to public school or go to see our family physician, we are consuming public goods. The identities of citizen and consumer come together, not without difficulty and even contradiction, when we use our roads, our hospitals, and our schools, or when we turn to the police for protection and safety. The important difference lies in what we can legitimately expect as "citizen-consumers" of public goods and what we can expect when, as private consumers, we buy for our enjoyment in the private marketplace.

Providers who supply public goods must serve collective as well as individual needs and meet different standards than firms that serve a private market. Consumers and suppliers exist in both worlds — the public as well as the private. But the two worlds are different: their values, their goals, their standards, their responsibilities, and their accountability create different spaces. When we consume private goods, we do so in the shadow of the marketplace, but when we consume public goods, we do so in the shadow of citizenship.[3] Private consumers consider only their own needs, but as citizen-consumers, we hope, we consider our own needs in the context of others. These differences are large and consequential.

The arguments between advocates of the market and defenders of the state are more than two centuries old, but they are taking on new shape as public markets develop in the post-industrial age. The label "citizen-consumer" has new meaning as citizens enter the market for public as well as private goods. Health care and education are public as well as private goods. The alarmed reaction to a single suspected case of Ebola in Ontario in February 2001 is vivid evidence of the obvious public benefit of health care: curing the individual provides benefit to all of us, as the spread of infectious disease is limited.

Although education and health care are both public goods, they differ in important ways. At least in theory, we can enjoy the process of becoming educated and the benefits of being educated for their own sake. Literacy can bring an intrinsic pleasure that is independent of the economic opportunities it creates. Reading a book can be one of life's pleasures, independent of the value of literacy as a life-skill. Health is also a joy — and a right — independent of any other opportunities it provides. With luck and sensible behaviour, however, most of us can enjoy being healthy without using health-care services on a regular basis. Health care, or the treatment of illness, is not a good that we voluntarily like to use for the sheer pleasure it provides. If coronary bypass surgery in a leading hospital were offered as a prize in a raffle, very few of us would buy a ticket. Many more might if the prize were a year's free education at a fine school.

There are also differences in the way we use these two public goods. To become educated, we generally must go to school on a regular basis. Participation in education usually stretches over many years, beginning at an early age, when parents make decisions on behalf of their children. Access to health care for many of us is a bumpier, more intermittent, and less continuous need than access to education. We can go for many years making very limited demands on the health-care system and then use it intensely for a restricted period of time. Health care as a public good brings with it much greater uncertainty than education, and it is this uncertainty that creates the need for insurance. Markets in education and health care mirror these differences in the nature of the two public goods.

A Public Cry of Alarm

It is worthwhile to look at public education and health care not only because they are intrinsically important public goods, but because they are high on the list of public worries. People are upset about public education and health care. Many of us are sounding a relentlessly alarmist tone: we now believe that two of our most important social institutions are broken and need to be fixed. Our worry about education and health care is not superficial. It strikes deeply at the way we think about public goods, the way we think about society, the way we think about government, and the way we think about ourselves. Our heated and often polemical discussion of education and health care is a barometer of far more basic currents that are coursing through the post-industrial age.

This public dissatisfaction is a stunning reversal from a decade ago, when Canadians were generally satisfied with health care and education and worried about the economy, employment, debt, and deficits. Canadians are now more likely than their counterparts in Britain, Australia, and the United States to agree that fundamental change in their health-care system is necessary. Education is also a serious concern. Less than half of the Canadian public is satisfied with the education their children are receiving. "For the public," as Allan Gregg succinctly puts it, "the quo has no status."[4]

It is no surprise that the Canadian public is badly divided about what has gone wrong and deeply ambivalent about how to fix education and health care. As we saw in chapter 2, institutions created during the industrial age and the modern welfare state fit less and less well with post-industrial societies in the making. Canadians are now more willing to look for solutions to markets, both private and public, and to the competition markets stimulate.

Across North America, parents and governments are looking to competition through school choice as a remedy for the ills of the public education system. Canadians also want to maintain their universal medical-care system, but only a small percentage are still willing to pay higher taxes to do so. A surprisingly large number of Canadians are now willing to consider some form of private funding

and delivery, if that is what it takes to preserve the system.[5] The shift in public opinion about health care is
particularly astonishing in a country that, for the past two
decades, identified its unique universal medical-care system as its greatest collective success. We were justifiably
proud of the fairness, the quality, and the efficiency of our
system, and smug when we looked at the inequity and
blatant unfairness of the medical-care system in the
United States, where 40 million Americans have no health
insurance at all.[6] Indeed, pride in the Canadian system of
universal health care became a defining component of
national identity. Something has gone seriously amiss.

Are Public Systems Failing?

Public schools have been savaged by stinging criticism in
the past two decades. A new emphasis on what students
know and what skills they have so that they can, as we
hear again and again, "better meet the challenges of the
post-industrial economy," infuses public talk about education. There is cause for concern. What students know
does matter in a global knowledge-based economy, and
the results from a dry-run standardized literacy test in
Ontario's public high schools in 2000 seemed disquieting:
more than one in four of Ontario's tenth grade students
failed the test.[7] Newspaper headlines across the province
shrieked, "Ontario's public schools are failing!"

These kinds of results have generated widespread
alarm across North America about the quality of education that the public system is delivering.[8] The critics
charge that Canadian schools are not providing the basic

knowledge that their graduates require either to prosper in the global economy or to contribute to civil society. Ignorance serves no agenda: not of economic liberals who want to fit knowledge and skills to the global economy, not of political liberals who believe passionately that the existence of a high-quality education is the most important building block of a civic democracy, and not of radical individualists who look at the whole child and want an education that is tailored to individual needs.[9]

Concern is also high in Britain, New Zealand, Australia, and the United States. Students in the United States did not do as well as those from other post-industrial countries on international achievement tests. The pace of reform in the U.S. has become frenetic: redesign of curricula, experimentation with new methods of teaching, additional spending, more rigorous standards of teacher certification. Then there was more homework, less homework, a return to basics, phonics, whole language, back to phonics, then core curricula followed by widespread choice of courses, followed by a reintroduction of core curricula. Over the past two decades, as performance has stagnated in the United States, per pupil spending has doubled, class size has shrunk, and teacher education has improved. It all seems to have made little difference; student performance on standardized tests still has not materially improved.

In Canada, the tone of public discussion is less apocalyptic and the pace of reform less frenetic, but as we have seen, worry about the quality of public schools has grown substantially among the public in the past five years.

Critics charge that our public schools are failing to improve the basic skills of students, that they are failing to meet the needs of poorer children in Canada, particularly among the First Nations, and that students are shockingly ignorant of Canadian history and culture. A disturbingly high proportion of students — as well as citizens — are unable to name Canada's first prime minister or identify seminal events in Canadian history.[10] Whatever the criterion — whether it is knowledge, or equity and justice, or democratic values — schools are failing.

Many of the same concerns about quality are threaded through our public conversation about health care. Added to them is deep worry about how governments across Canada will pay for growing demands for the expansion of medicare beyond hospitals and doctors. In Canada, public spending on health care generally consumes a much larger proportion of provincial budgets than does education, and after five years of constraint in the mid-1990s, spending is growing again.[11] Some allege that it is escalating out of control. As the Fyke Commission in Saskatchewan (the birthplace of medicare) recently warned, even if no new responsibilities are added to the current universal medical-care system, the government is still locked into spending almost all of its forecast increase in revenues on health care.[12]

The financial challenge is clear: if present trends continue and the tax base remains relatively constant, spending on health care threatens to compromise other public goods that governments across Canada provide. Premier Mike Harris of Ontario recently concluded that the current universal health-care system is not sustainable. Even if this conclusion is overly alarmist, and some argue that it is, the financial imperative for change in the health-care system is clear.

The crisis is not restricted only to the growing costs of the health care that is currently available. Canadians complain that not enough is available, and what is available is often not available quickly enough. Medicare covers Canadians only for medically necessary services, and over the past three decades, medical practice has changed. Hospital stays are now much shorter, a great deal of surgery is done on an outpatient basis, and patients go home earlier, needing care and medication at home. New drugs are available that make it possible at times to avoid hospitalization entirely, but drugs outside the hospital are not necessarily covered by public insurance. To use economic language for a moment, the demand for new kinds of health care is growing and the supply that is available is becoming more expensive every year. Canada's health-care system, concludes one recent analysis, "is in a straightjacket."[13] Escalating costs and growing demand — for the expansion of health-care coverage, for shorter waiting times and waiting lists, and for more effective care — fuel the calls for efficiency.

The Contested Causes: Why Are Schools and Health Care "Failing"?

What makes a school — and a school system — effective? Until we answer that question, any calculation of efficiency, or cost-effectiveness, is logically and practically nonsense. To urge schools to become more efficient when there is no understanding of what makes a school effective is to use the language of a cult. Not surprisingly, there is fierce debate about what makes a school effective.

The strongest determinant of student achievement globally is the socio-economic status of the family. Indeed, this may account for as much as half of student performance. The socio-economic status of the family is a major influence at home, where parents establish basic educational values and work habits, and at school, where children bring their values and attitudes with them.[14]

Yet some schools are clearly more effective than others, even when the socio-economic status of families is relatively similar. At Joliette High School, in a small town northeast of Montreal, Quebec, 190 students come from struggling families with below-average incomes. A quarter of the children live in homes where neither parent has a full-time job or a high-school diploma. The school is modest, without much of the new equipment that bigger schools in larger cities have. And yet students achieved results in provincial exams in 1999 that placed Joliette among the top 15 percent in the province, matching, and in some cases surpassing, private schools. "In a lot of schools," explained one fifteen-year-old student, "look at the students. The lower their mark, the cooler they are. Here, we all want to do well in life and pass with good marks."[15]

Critics disagree, often strongly, about why so few public schools are effective. The most trenchant — and radical — critiques locate their ineffectiveness not in the schools

themselves, but in the broader public institutions that created and now manage the public school system. Our
current public education system, they insist, is a creature
of the industrial age, designed at the turn of the last century and still with us today.[16] The same reformers who
pushed for efficiency through merit-based bureaucracies
and rational planning ended local autonomy and created
a large bureaucratic professional public educational system. It was, in the language of the times, the "one best
system": experts, professionals, and bureaucrats knew
what kind of education students needed and how it could
best be provided.[17] Drained out of education was the local
difference and diversity so characteristic of pre-industrial
schooling. It is in this sense that the "one best system" is a
factory model: the organization — if not the content — of
public education was standardized, homogenized, and
delivered as a mass-market public good.

This "one best" model was a comfortable fit with
industrial economies and societies, and with their politics. It fits very uneasily with post-industrial economies
that privilege innovation and differentiation, and
operate through flexible networks rather than command-
and-control hierarchies. It fits even less well with values
of autonomy and self-expression, and with the prevail-
ing attitude of deep scepticism toward government. The
"one best" model fits increasingly less easily with a state
that contracts out and partners rather than microman-
ages and directly delivers programs, as the industrial
state did. As economies and societies became post-
industrial, it is no coincidence that the next wave of

critics demanded radical restructuring of the school system, not by changing the content of what is taught or by
changing the way students are taught, but by changing
the governing institutions — again, in the name of
efficiency.

Canadians are also worried — seriously worried —
that their health-care system is not sustainable. When the
fundamentals of Canada's universal public insurance for
medically necessary services were put in place, equality
of access was the most important goal. Political leaders
and the public expected that public revenues would be
adequate to sustain the system, and indeed, the evidence
was encouraging. A bilateral monopoly of governments
and physicians set prices for insured services. This should
have been a classic opportunity for price-fixing, cost esca-
lation, and inefficiency.

But that is not what happened. Canada controlled
costs better than the U.S., with its unregulated market
and insurance only for the very poor and the elderly.
Between 1971 and 1985, the real fees of physicians
declined in Canada while they rose in the United States. It
appears that a public system of medical insurance was
better at cost-containment than private markets. The
practice of medicine also seemed to be more internally
efficient in Canada than it was in the United States: office
expenses for physicians as a proportion of gross billings
were significantly lower in Canada than they were for
their counterparts in the United States.[18]

Only in the late 1980s, as concern about the growing
deficit and cumulative public debt began to grow, did

political attention turn to controlling the costs of health care. Efficiency, often invoked in public discussion, was defined narrowly as cost-containment. From 1992 through 1997, per capita public expenditures for health care not only held stable, but dropped. Expenditure did not keep pace with population growth, much less allow for the added costs associated with the aging of the population and new technologies.[19] Controlling — or cutting — costs can be inefficient if it reduces the effectiveness of health care by an even larger margin. Much of the language of the past decade misconstrues efficiency to mean cost-containment. When this happens, as I argued in the previous chapter, efficiency becomes a cult.

It has been the almost exclusive emphasis on efficiency as cost-containment that has undermined any meaningful reform of the medical-care system. To oversimplify only a little, Canada has had neither reform nor serious examination of the cost-effectiveness of the system, but only cost-containment by provincial and federal governments seeking desperately to control their budgets. Governments generally did not ask how *effective* medical care was in relation to its costs; they asked only how *much* it cost.

It is no surprise that after a decade of cost-containment, the effectiveness and the sustainability of the health-care system are now the subject of serious concern. Canadians worry that the delisting of services, early discharge from public institutions, and the escalating costs of drugs threaten the benefits that they receive. We worry about our access to home care and long-term care

as the medical component of health care shrinks. And we
worry about the quality of the medical care we receive, as
well as our access to timely care, as cost-containment and
cost-cutting constrain the medical system. As a task force
on health policy concluded, "Canadians on waiting lists
are not imagining their anxieties."[20] These worries have
created a crisis in public confidence. Public attention is
now increasingly focused not only on costs, but also
explicitly on effectiveness and quality.

One solution many Canadians are looking at today, a
solution that would have been unthinkable even five
years ago, is public funding of providers that work outside a framework of universal access. Vouchers in
education and medical savings accounts for health care
are two such proposals that would allow public funding
to follow citizen-consumers to those providers. Citizens
can shop for education and health care wherever they
want. How does this work? Are these markets more efficient than the public system? What story do vouchers,
two-tier medicine, and medical savings accounts tell us
about the funding of public goods outside a framework of
universal access?

Education

Thomas Paine, writing two centuries ago, first proposed
school vouchers as a strategy for the radical reform of the
institutional structure of education. Paine recommended
that governments pay, "as a remission of taxes, to every
poor family, out of the surplus taxes . . . four pounds
a year for every child under fourteen years of age;

enjoining the parents of such children to send them to school, to learn reading, writing, and common arithmetic; the ministers of every parish, of every denomination, to certify jointly to an office, for that purpose, that this duty is performed."[21]

The argument is deceptively simple and by now familiar: create a market for public education by giving parents vouchers to spend at a private school of their choice; treat parents and their children as individual "consumers," educators as "suppliers," and government as the regulator of the rules of the market, not as the direct provider of public education. Through competition, the market will ignite a race to the top, and hold the ineffi cient accountable.[22]

Why create a market that allows public funds to flow to private providers outside the public system? Proponents of vouchers put forward two somewhat different arguments. Economic liberals look at the state as the sole supplier of primary and secondary education and cry, "Monopoly!" A monopoly market, they charge, creates all kinds of inefficiencies and has no built-in checks to assure quality.[23] Alternatively, they argue, an educational market will foster competition among schools, rewarding the cost-effective schools that provide quality education and punishing the failures as parents "exit." Parents will withdraw their children from schools that do not achieve results and use their vouchers elsewhere, and schools that are unable to attract enough "customers" for the services they provide will be forced to close. The introduction of "market-like" thinking and the threat of "exit" will encourage all schools within the public system to provide education that responds to parents' concerns and does so efficiently.

Others look at politics rather than economics when they excoriate the ineffectiveness, and therefore the inefficiency, of public education. They argue that state bureaucracies are captured by political constituencies — teachers' unions and professional educators — and primarily serve their interests. The educational system is too constrained to make meaningful improvement in the quality of the education that it delivers; the arterial sclerosis of bureaucracy is too advanced to reverse, much less to cure. "Bureaucracy," as John Chubb and Terry Moe put it, "is unambiguously bad for school organization."[24] The solution is to change radically the institutional structure that delivers education.

The argument for vouchers is not restricted to the ineffectiveness of public education, but also extends to its transparent inequalities. The current public education system, critics allege, is inefficient at providing equality. Proponents of vouchers argue that families living in inner cities cannot afford either to buy private education or to move to neighbourhoods whose public schools provide higher-quality education. Their children are trapped in failing schools. The argument applies as much to Manila as it does to Milwaukee, as much to Santiago as it does to San Francisco, and as much to Taipei as it does to Toronto.[25] Publicly financed education systems are often of low quality in the poorest neighbourhoods, partly as a result of funding from an inadequate tax base and partly as a consequence of internal inefficiency. Yet families have no choice but to continue to send their children to these schools. Visiting a school in the poorest section of Cairo, or Santiago, or Winnipeg makes transparently clear how serious an argument this is and how much of our consideration it deserves.

The political and the economic arguments reinforce each other. To put bluntly the point of the proponents of vouchers: a monopoly that is captured by special interests, and is responsive — if it is responsive at all — to those best able to voice their interests, is unlikely to provide quality and equal access to public education. The system, proponents of school choice argue, is truly broken, and it cannot be fixed by increased spending or tampering with mechanics.

A look at what has happened when vouchers have been tried is the best way to get beneath the sound and fury of the polemics. The best-known experiment with vouchers began in Milwaukee. The goal of the voucher program was clear: it was explicitly designed to provide better educational opportunities to the children of poor families. It was founded by an African-American state representative, Annette "Polly" Williams, a liberal Democrat, and ultimately supported by Governor Tommy Thompson, a conservative Republican. It is easy to understand how these two radically different political agendas crossed ideological lines and converged: the growth of inner-city segregation in Milwaukee had led to a desegregation order in 1976, forced busing, extensive white flight to the suburbs, and an increase in private-school enrolment by families who could afford to pay the fees and chose not to move. In Milwaukee, as in many other large cities in the United States, as one analyst of the schools put it, there were "two worlds of education separated by a few miles."[26]

The experimental voucher program adopted by Milwaukee in 1990 was targeted and limited, with built-in safeguards. Only families with incomes to 175 percent of the poverty line or lower were eligible; current students in private schools were ineligible; and voucher students had to be randomly selected so that schools could not "cream-skim" or select only the best students. It was a program of affirmative action through markets.

Did the Milwaukee program work? What did the voucher program accomplish? The record is mixed, and surprising. The program was not more cost-effective, but it significantly improved equitable access to education. These results are not what either advocates of the market or defenders of the state would expect.

On the cost side of the equation, there were few, if any, gains from the voucher program in Milwaukee. Generally, vouchers did not reduce costs.[27] But the failure to reduce costs does not make the Milwaukee program inefficient. If the private schools that accepted voucher students were generally more effective, if they produced higher levels of achievement among their students while holding costs pretty well constant, then an argument can still be made for efficiency. Although the story is contested, and far from over, it is mixed: some voucher students did significantly better, but many others did no better at all. On both dimensions of efficiency — cost and effectiveness — there is little hard evidence that voucher students did significantly better than those who stayed in the public schools.[28] Defenders of markets would be disappointed.

The story is very different when we look at equity. The Milwaukee program provided significant opportunity for students from low-income families to exit from public schools, giving them much more equitable access to education. The signal success of public funding of private institutions comes in greater efficiency at promoting equity, but only when the funding is restricted and targeted. Critics of markets have often pointed to the inequalities that competition generates. The paradoxical result of a restricted market is not what they would expect.

The Milwaukee program improved equity only because vouchers were restricted and targeted. When vouchers were given to everyone — as they were earlier in Chile and subsequently in Cleveland — they sharply reinforced inequality: current private-school users consumed most of the vouchers. Vouchers in Chile and Cleveland were inefficient at improving equity. On the contrary, permitting public funding to flow with no restrictions compounded inequities. This is exactly what critics of markets would expect and defenders would acknowledge.

The story of public funds flowing to private schools is that it provides real gains only when programs are restricted. But restricting vouchers raises large social questions. Social dilemmas grow out of the consequences of individual decisions for the larger whole. Students who remain in the poorest schools lose their most articulate champions for change and improvement: when the most highly motivated parents exit, those who stay are deprived of their most articulate voices. Here the citizen-consumer differs from the private consumer. How much opportunity for an individual student from a low-income family should be sacrificed for the sake of other students who stay in their local public school? How long should the students who are prepared to leave for a private school be asked to wait for their local public school to improve? These are hard questions with no easy answers.

Restrictions on the public funds that flow to private providers create other social dilemmas. They are a form of means-testing that historically has created social stereotyping. Voucher students could become stigmatized, and political support for voucher programs could evaporate. Targeted programs are also likely to engender resentment among those who are not eligible: parents who are dissatisfied with their local schools but do not qualify for a voucher because their income is just above the line. Usually, these parents cannot afford to pay the fees for private schooling. This group is fairly large and politically important across North America. It is precisely this political dynamic that pushes the creation of universal, rather than targeted, voucher programs, with pernicious consequences for equity.

International experiments — and experience — have come home to Canada. The government of Ontario is about to introduce the first voucher-like program in public education. It recently passed legislation that will extend tax credits of up to $3,500 for any child to attend private schools.[29] "The tax credits," argues William Robson of the C. D. Howe Institute, "provide a much greater degree of choice for parents to elect the schools that provide them with the services that they need."[30] But which parents? Only those parents who can afford to pay the balance of the fees will be able to take advantage of the credit. Public funds will flow to private institutions in a way that will systematically discriminate against poorer families.

Ontario has introduced the tax credit, the equivalent of a voucher, at a time when it has imposed new standards of effectiveness in the public system, but the private schools are exempt from any testing of effectiveness until the ninth grade. It is impossible to conclude that such a program is cost-effective, given the absence of any information on the effectiveness of private schools at the primary level. "What we will have now," argues the president of the Ontario Secondary School Teachers' Federation (admittedly not a disinterested party), "is a two-tier education system supported by tax dollars with two-tier accountability."[31]

There is real irony here. Governments are now prepared to use public money to subsidize parents to remove their children from the curriculum that they have imposed in the public schools and that they insist is more effective. In Canada, England, Wales, Northern Ireland, and New Zealand, governments have imposed more and more stringent curriculum requirements. They have restricted choice by students of what they learn in order to increase what they know. Parents have less and less choice about the knowledge and skills acquired by their children in the public school system. At the same time, these governments have introduced choice of school, by enabling "exit" from the public system, in order to improve efficiency in the delivery of education. This is a very curious concept of school choice.[32]

Health Care

Vouchers in public education are only one experiment in directing public funding to private providers outside the public system. In health care, Canadians are now talking about two other systems that would also allow public money to flow outside the public system. One is long familiar to Canadians: two-tier medicine, in which the private system is indirectly supported by the public system. The second is more radical and as yet untried: medical savings accounts, which would work much like vouchers in public education. How would these experiments live? What underpins the new shape of the conversation about health care?

Mention of two-tier medicine has traditionally been a lightning rod across Canada. Until very recently, any discussion of a parallel private system was politically impermissible. Even the suspicion that a government was toying with the concept provoked a firestorm. Canada is unique: it has the only publicly insured medical-care system where patients generally cannot, even if they so choose, pay for private medical care for insured services. But Canadians do pay — directly or through private insurance — for health-care services that are not considered medically necessary.[33]

Proponents of a two-tier medical system work from market logic. They argue that a second tier would provide a much-needed shock to the public system. It would create a more competitive environment. David Gratzer, a leading critic of medicare, argues that a privately financed parallel system could "be the Federal Express method of health-care reform — by direct comparison, the courier forces the post office to be more accountable."[34] The reasoning is flawed: two-tier medicine would provide this kind of shock if — and only if — the private system had to provide a full range of care for all patients and not just cream off the relatively healthy and wealthy.

The arguments against a two-tier medical system have been well rehearsed in Canada. The pre-eminent argument, of course, focuses on the increase in inequity that is the inevitable consequence of a health-care system that is not committed to universal access. If there were no differences in the quality of care or the timeliness of access between the public and private systems, people would not be willing to pay the substantial premiums for private care. The private system thrives by differentiating itself from the public system — by increasing the inequities. To put the argument bluntly, to survive, a parallel private system must provide markedly superior health care for those who can afford to pay. Inequity is an inevitable consequence.

If the second tier were truly private, then we could argue that those who wish to pay for "better" health care — whatever that is — should be free to do so. Why should people be restricted, the argument goes, from spending their money as they please? Very rarely, however, is a parallel private system truly "private." Health-care systems where doctors are allowed to work in both the public and the private sectors blur the lines between the two. Doctors and other health-care workers are trained largely at public expense; the cost of their training acts as a public subsidy to a private system. The public system in effect subsidizes the private.

Doctors who work in both sectors are also logically driven to steer patients who can afford the fees from the public to the private system. Physicians have a strong incentive to privilege the private over the public system so that those patients who can afford to pay continue to seek care privately. Those they target are the wealthy, not the poor. The most highly skilled physicians will tend to spend more time in the private system, and gradually the public system will become less, not more, cost-effective. A well-functioning private system depends on a weak public system.[35] This kind of perverse incentive structure leads to a less, not more, efficient public system, as well as far more inequitable access to quality care.

Proponents of a two-tier system tend to argue from market logic. Markets are only efficient, however, when they are genuinely competitive and inefficient suppliers can be forced out of business. The structure of a two-tier health-care system where physicians can work in both vitiates that logic: providers are guaranteed a "floor price" by the public system, but there is no ceiling on what they can charge privately. Teachers are not allowed to work simultaneously in both a private and a public school, where they are free to give less attention to the public school and steer students to the private instution. Yet this is what has happened in Britain's health-care system, and in many other health-care systems around the world. When health-care providers work in both systems, they get at least the price that would be paid by the publicly funded system, as well as the bonus provided by the private charges. Again, the logic is perverse: the total spent on health care rises — because of the bonus — and providers cannot be forced out of the market. This is hardly conducive to efficiency, the principal promise of a private parallel market.[36] Two-tier medicine is inefficient at being inequitable.

How well do these arguments stand up? The United Kingdom and New Zealand both have two-tier systems. Waiting lists in the public system, one of the most important concerns Canadians have, are proportionately longer in these two countries than they are in Canada.[37] The availability of private care does not relieve the pressure on the public system. Two-tier systems are clearly not the solution; they do not provide the efficiency that advocates of markets claim.

A far more radical proposal puts purchasing power directly in the hands of patients, or health-care consumers. It would impose no restrictions on the flow of public funding. Indeed, the proposal for medical savings accounts would abolish the distinction between private and public delivery of health care. This proposal is akin in spirit to vouchers in the education system: with vouchers, dollars follow students, and with medical savings accounts, dollars would follow patients. We could shop for our health care wherever we like.

Where would we get the money to shop for health care? We would each receive a direct grant, adjusted for age, gender, and health status, from our government each year; this would be deposited in a special savings account. This account would cover the routine range of illnesses, and we would draw on it to pay the health-care provider of our choice. We would also be covered by catastrophic insurance to protect against major illnesses. Proposals for medical savings accounts vary in the details, but they are all built on two key pillars: the direct transfer of funds, which people are free to spend as they choose on health care across the continuum — from disease prevention to health care; and catastrophic insurance.[38]

The logic of the plan is simple. For routine health-care expenses, we pay directly from our medical savings account. When that account is exhausted, we pay out of our own pockets up to a predetermined level. It is this gap between the amount allotted for routine care and cat- astrophic coverage — the equivalent of an annual user fee — that lays bare the underlying logic. Through unlimited choice and user fees, we become responsible for our health-care choices.[39] Patients as citizen-consumers of health care are both free to make choices and responsible for their choices.

Not only would citizen-consumers become more responsible, the argument continues, but those who provide health-care would become more efficient. This kind of plan would end all direct spending on health-care institutions. Governments or health authorities would give no more block grants to hospitals. Hospitals and all other health-care institutions would be dependent on whatever market share they could attract, and they would compete for patients in the marketplace. They would want to invest in the latest technologies in order to improve the quality of their services to enhance their capacity to compete. Resources would naturally flow to the most efficient. A publicly financed market, supplemented by insurance, would be created across the continuum of health care, and institutions and providers would respond by becoming more cost-effective.

Advocates of medical savings accounts also expect to see changes in the way primary-care (or family) physicians behave. The current fee-for-service system, they allege, leads primary-care doctors to rush patients through their offices and to overuse diagnostic testing and prescription drugs. Doctors currently are motivated to see as many patients as they can, as quickly as they can. The most popular remedy for this problem within the current system is a proposal to group together primary-care providers — doctors, nurses, and other health-care professionals — to provide around-the-clock service to patients within a region. Physicians would be paid for the type of patient they see — age, gender, and health risk — regardless of how many times they see that patient within a year. Advocates of voucher-like medical savings accounts argue that this solution would only deepen the problems of the current medical-care system; it would reduce physicians' incentives to be productive. Medical savings accounts, they promise, would encourage doctors to be competitive and efficient.

The argument for medical savings accounts sounds seductive. Its language is that of choice, autonomy, and responsibility, the language increasingly spoken by citizens in the post-industrial age. The state is no longer manager, but instead becomes the regulator of quality and standards, a fit with the new face it increasingly shows to citizens. Health-care providers compete, and efficiency improves. Although the language is seductive, unfortunately the argument is logically flawed.

The logic of medical savings accounts depends critically on the capacity to provide catastrophic insurance. If account holders could turn to publicly funded insurance that insured everyone, the health-care system would respond to the same kinds of incentives that are now in place. The incentive for citizen-consumers to be responsible and for health-care providers to compete — the defining elements in market logic — would be diminished by the knowledge that public insurance was waiting in the wings. Citizens would have to be responsible only until their insurance coverage began, and health-care providers would compete to spend publicly funded insurance payments. This is a very weak version of market logic.

That is not the only problem that publicly funded

insurance would encounter. The public funder would almost completely lose its capacity to control costs. In Singapore, the government created an arm's-length agency to run medical savings accounts. It is no accident that the agency refuses to sell catastrophic coverage to the disabled, to anyone older than seventy-five, or to anyone with severe pre-existing conditions. This is a very curious kind of universal plan that denies coverage to those who need it most. The plan in Singapore also carefully limits its potential liability.[40] In this kind of system, any one of us with a chronic or severe illness would quickly exhaust our lifetime coverage.[41]

If universal public insurance does not cover those who need it most under a system of medical savings accounts, then private insurance markets are the only logical alternative. Private insurance companies are traditionally wary of high costs and uncertain needs — precisely the characteristics of catastrophic illness. They routinely risk-rate people according to age, disability, and lifestyle, and avoid those individuals they consider to be high risk. If you have applied for health insurance for travel outside Canada recently, you know exactly what I mean. Yet it is precisely the highest-risk who are most likely to need catastrophic insurance. For the most vulnerable among the population, the result is an inordinately high premium or no coverage at all. A private market for catastrophic insurance would discriminate strongly against those who need insurance coverage most.

The similarity between educational vouchers and medical savings accounts goes only so far. Educational vouchers do not need to be backed up by insurance, and they can be relatively uniform because the costs of educating a student within the public system do not vary widely and are predictable. The costs of health-care services for an individual patient are neither consistent nor predictable. Medical vouchers depend on insurance, and for anybody but a public insurer committed to universal access, the incentive to avoid high-risk patients is overwhelming.[42]

Those who propose vouchers for public education and health care couch what they say in the language of efficiency. But they also speak the discourse of choice, autonomy, and individual responsibility — the language of more and more citizens in post-industrial society. Proponents of voucher programs in education also draw on a language that is only now beginning to be heard: choice as a fundamental right of citizens. Governor Tommy Thompson of Wisconsin put it explicitly: "School choice is more than a program . . . it is a philosophy. It is a belief that poor parents have the same *right to choose* that other parents do. . . . That's education serving the public!"[43]

The stories that vouchers in health care and education tell in practice are different from what they promise. A publicly funded voucher program for health care that is critically dependent on private insurance markets offers little promise when universal health care is the public good. It is not more cost-effective, and it is dramatically less efficient at providing equity. Educational vouchers tell a more complex story. When they are universal, they deliver neither greater cost-effectiveness nor greater equity. When they are targeted at low-income families, they do offer significant opportunities for students to move to better schools. Above all, parents of voucher students are significantly more satisfied with their children's education. When we are evaluating targeted voucher programs in education, the debate is not about efficiency at all. It is about the larger collective responsibility to provide opportunity to children of low-income families — and their right to choose. This is a conversation worth having.

Public Markets in Education: Efficiency, Choice, and Community

Allowing public funding to flow to private institutions outside a framework of universal access is one way of blending markets and states. But it is not very promising. Restricting public funding to providers that work only in the public system may have greater potential. This is a more truly public market, with a clear commitment to universality but with underlying market logic. In this kind of market, the providers of public goods are still separate from the purchasers, from those who fund public goods. Providers are then encouraged to compete for public funds, and out of competition comes efficiency.

Public markets play out somewhat differently in education and health care. In education, they are built around charter schools, with public funding going only to schools within the public system. States that permit charter schools allow citizens to establish independent schools and then expect these schools to compete for students. Funding goes not directly to the parents, but to the school. In health care, Britain has experimented most extensively in the past fifteen years with public markets; these markets clearly separate those who are charged with buying health care from those who supply care, in order to stimulate competition. The money goes not to patients, but to health-care institutions and providers that compete for public funding. Those institutions that buy care on behalf of the state look for the most cost-effective care available and reward the efficient.

The creation of public markets within the public system is the most significant change in the face of the state since the creation of merit-based bureaucracies to manage the delivery of public goods a hundred years ago. How have these experiments worked? Do public markets deliver the efficiency they promise? Do they provide other unanticipated advantages and disadvantages? What happens to the citizen-consumer who can shop only in public space?

We begin with a look at charter schools. First, what is a charter school? It is an independent public school of choice, firmly embedded in the public system, accountable for its results, but freed as much as possible from rules about the way it teaches. The first charter law was enacted in Minnesota in 1991, and today there are more than 1,700 charter schools, with more than half a million students in thirty-one states in the United States. Alberta passed the first charter legislation in Canada in 1994, allowing a maximum of fifteen charters throughout the province. Thus far, against the considerable opposition of local school boards, Alberta has chartered twelve schools.

Why are charter schools created? They are generally set up by educators or parents who are dissatisfied with their existing public schools and wish to provide a different educational environment or a different kind of education than is publicly available. The diversity of goals reflects the breadth of the charter-school movement, as well as the differences in socio-economic status and cultural background of those who found charter schools. In Alberta, for example, two charter schools target gifted children, one focuses on children whose first language is not English, one focuses on "at risk" teens, several stress a structured learning environment, one combines basic education with an enriched music curriculum, and the newest school focuses on science education. Generally, the most important goals are improving educational achievement, increasing personal safety for students, and building community.

How are these schools created? Founders must get approval from their local school or provincial or state board. Once they are chartered, they receive the basic level of per pupil funding allocated to regular public schools for every student they enrol. Their charter is reviewed every three to five years, and at least in theory, charter schools can be closed if they fail to meet expectations.[44] Charter schools are generally accountable to governments or to the local school boards that issued the charter. They are responsible for results, but they are free to produce these results as they think best. They are not

obligated to follow the regulations of education departments in the way they deliver the curriculum, nor are
they required to hire unionized or certified staff. Charter
schools are "tight as to ends, but loose as to means."[45] The
emphasis is on transparency and outcomes, not on
process.

Are charter schools effective? Effective at what? They
clearly are satisfying parents. Surveys show consistently
high parent satisfaction, and 70 percent of charter schools
report that they have waiting lists.[46] If parent satisfaction
with their children's schools is one measure of effectiveness — and not an unimportant measure — charter
schools can be considered more effective than their counterparts in the public system.

What about effectiveness in increasing educational
achievement? It is still early, but the evidence on student
achievement suggests that charter schools are not
performing very differently from public schools. In
Los Angeles, in comparison to schools serving similar
children, several charter schools were able to improve
student performance significantly. In Alberta, performance results on provincial measures of learning show that
students in charter schools are generally achieving "at
least as well" as students in public schools.[47] Generally,
however, charter schools have yet to demonstrate the
capacity to increase student achievement through more
effective practices. Charter schools, as an astute analyst of
the charter movement concludes, are scoring high on
process and low on results.[48] If effectiveness is defined as
improving student achievement at roughly the same cost

as the public system, the claim for greater efficiency of charter schools is hard to substantiate.

Are charter schools efficient at improving equity? Here, too, the evidence is mixed. Charter schools unquestionably have discretion, subject to the terms of their charter and government legislation, over the individual students they accept. By quietly rejecting applications, schools can actively seek out the best students and reject at-risk students who will be far more expensive to educate and may reduce the school's performance record. As the director of the Valley Charter School near San Francisco confided, "If a parent with a handicapped child knocks on my door, I politely urge her to visit the next public school down the road."[49] Charter schools can easily engage in "cream skimming" of the best students.

Yet minorities in the United States — particularly African Americans and Hispanic Americans — are often strong supporters of charter schools, which provide an exit from public schools that are not meeting their children's needs. More African Americans support school vouchers than oppose them, and they consistently support vouchers more strongly than does the white population. Their endorsement of vouchers is evidence of how dissatisifed they are with their schools and how strongly they reject the status quo.[50] They argue that powerful educational bureaucracies, responsive largely to the strongest political constituencies, do not adequately serve the needs of less powerful minorities. Many charter schools primarily serve students from minority communities.

The strongest benefit of charter schools may be in their capacity to build community, an important resource that mediates the impact of social class on achievement. In the past century, schools became increasingly divorced from community control. "The public as a real force in the life of schools was deliberately and systematically rooted out," argues David Matthews, president of the Kettering Foundation. "Citizens were replaced with a new group of professionals, true guardians of the public interest, there to do what it was assumed citizens couldn't or shouldn't do."[51] As thousands of small schools were consolidated into larger districts and larger boards, with an emphasis on expertise, orderly management, uniform operations, and large-scale organizations, local control and community engagement were further eroded.[52] The one best system — the factory model — is no friend to civic engagement and community.

Surprisingly, market imperatives reinforce community building. By expanding the choices parents have in education, social capital and civic engagement grow.[53] The reciprocal connections between engagement, trust, and education are interesting — and important. The greater the social capital in a community, the higher the level of trust and expectations of reciprocity among citizens, the more often parents come together voluntarily to work for public purposes, the better students perform. Coming together to found, organize, and sustain a charter school increases citizen engagement around a public good. Here, individual choice promotes collective, as well as individual, benefit. The process of building a charter school forges community ties that in turn sustain the school and improve the performance of children in the school. The community builds the school and the school builds the community. The development of local community and culture fits, paradoxically, with the market imperative to define and provide customized products for niche markets. Charter schools, operating in a public market, must attract parents and students, in part by clearly establishing their identity and market niche.

Unfortunately, it is not difficult to imagine how a larger charter-school movement could contribute to ethnic or racial segregation.[54] Schools can define the requirements of the curriculum in community terms and make it uncomfortable for students who come from different traditions. Almost half of all charter schools serve predominantly students who speak English as their first language, one-quarter serve mainly students who are visible minorities, and one-third have a significantly lower percentage of white students than other schools in their district.[55] The imperatives of the educational public market push toward product differentiation, rather than toward tolerance and inclusiveness. And the evidence is strong that parents do give weight to the kind of subcommunity in which they wish their children to be socialized. Many charter schools are indeed niche schools that appeal to communities with homogeneous values.

This is a troubling pattern. It is troubling for many who see the public school as a unique place where children from all backgrounds come together to share common experiences, create collective memories, learn a common vocabulary, and develop democratic values. The local community and culture that charter schools strengthen is not the vision of Horace Mann and the common-school advocates of the nineteenth century, or that of John Dewey and the progressive educators early in the twentieth century.[56] They hoped not that parents would withdraw from public space to protect their own community, but that parents from diverse communities would come together to agree on how the common school could be constructed in a democratic society to educate citizens for a civic society. The common school, however, is not serving some of its minorities well. The real threat to civic society, argue two observers of American democracy, lies in "the absence of civic engagement and in the standardization of the civic idea," not in the existence of multiple civic ideals.[57]

The fundamental causes of low student performance are persistent inequalities in school financing and stubbornly high rates of child poverty. As the communitarian impulse for charter schools grows, and political pressure for more funding for radically decentralized schools increases, support for the state in its attack on these causes of poor performance diminishes. The constituencies that traditionally supported a strong state, a state which could attack the inequalities that drive poor student performance, are now increasingly supporting radical decentralization of education and charter schools. Recent polls show growing support for charter schools among Latino and African-American parents, the populations now in the majority in many large cities in the

United States. They have given up on "voice" and prefer "exit" from existing public schools. "The retreat into our own schoolhouses . . . may be good for local community building," Bruce Fuller argues, "but it denies the fact that only in a larger public square can the structural (cross-community) causes of inequality be addressed."[58] Public markets in education raise hard questions, with no easy answers.

How can we explain the support for public markets in education, even though these markets have yet to fulfil their promise? The value of diversity has taken on new meaning in the age of the global economy. Individual choice and community have both become more important as sweeping global forces and an increasing distrust of government stoke the demand for autonomy, community, and accountability — as well as for knowledge. Schools that define themselves by their differences from the broad public are an easy fit with post-industrial social organization, where there are fewer shared beliefs and cultural references, and where citizens are less deferential to government. In this context, the communitarian impulse of charter schools becomes especially appealing.[59]

Although support for charter schools is growing, they still educate only a small minority of students in the landscape of public education. Nevertheless, the impact of the charter movement is rippling through public education as charter schools challenge the legitimacy of the existing system and increase the political pressure for choice within the public system. Charter schools are a way, insists one analyst of public education, to "inject market forces . . . into what many perceive as an over-regulated, over-centralized public education monopoly with strong allegiance to the status quo and no institutional imperative to improve student performance."[60] "The market," conclude others, "can surely inject dynamism and enterprise, while lubricating the engines of reform."[61]

It is paradoxical that the expansion of choice within the public system does not reduce the need for government. Charter schools change the role of government, but they do not decrease its importance. Those charter schools that have succeeded have built close relationships with their local or state education departments, as well as with private benefactors. "The escape to freedom," concludes one analyst of the charter experiment, "so eagerly sought by charter pioneers, often leaves behind the necessary resources and support. . . . Radical decentralization may become effective only if central agencies lend a hand."[62] It is no small irony that public markets in education need governments if they are to provide space for individual choice and community.

Universal Health Care: Efficiency or Choice?

Public markets are attractive not only in education, but in health care as well. Governments, we have seen, are worrying about costs, and the public is paying particular attention to effectiveness. In post-industrial societies, people are generally less deferential and more protective of choice. In Canada, if we create public markets in health care, we are likely to have less, not more, choice than we currently have. There is an intriguing irony here: public markets — which are built on choice — are the chosen instruments to preserve equity, but these kinds of markets would reduce the choice that citizen-consumers of health care in Canada currently have. They constrain choice because they authorize others to act on our behalf to purchase care. We would be able to choose only those who make the choice for us; we could no longer directly make the choice ourselves. This paradox of public markets as a constraint on choice deserves attention.

Canadians endured a painful process of public cost-cutting in the mid-1990s, cost-cutting that was preceded by years of constantly increasing deficits. As citizens, we are generally unwilling to run public deficits again, nor do we look favourably on higher taxes to support the growing demand for new kinds of publicly insured health-care services. Accustomed both to choice and universal access to medically necessary services, we are receptive to a language of efficiency. Efficiency matters — not as an end, but as a means — if choice and equity are both to be preserved.

Many critics argue that tinkering with Canada's health-care system to create greater efficiency — by targeting funding, through the kind of cost shifting from public institutions to families and individuals that has occurred over the past decade — will simply not work. Nor is it equitable. The answer some propose is to change the way funds are allocated to create a public market that separates the purchase of health care from the providers. The driving force of change is to enhance cost-effectiveness, and the solution is to create public markets that can increase efficiency.

Public markets are designed to promote competition among health-care providers without threatening equity. Proponents claim that public markets allow a public system to deliver health care efficiently within an overall cost ceiling that is established through the political process. How much money should go to health, one of several public goods in the basket? Citizens, through their political leaders, determine what share of public monies should be devoted to health promotion and health care. Once this judgement is made, public markets then work to ensure that these resources go where they are most needed within the health-care system.[63] These kinds of markets are an attempt not to reduce government spending on health care, but to increase efficiency in the allocation of resources across the system.[64] They are designed to introduce competition into the public sector, and to make sure that resources go where they are most needed.

Public markets vary. Today, Canada uses a mixed model to allocate resources. Provinces already allocate some resources through quasi-markets. The funding goes to physicians who attract patients — the money follows the choices of patients — and it is here that we have unlimited choice. Provincial governments generally use a more centrally planned system to allocate funds to hospitals through block funding; here, patients follow the money. Most proposals for public markets in health care mix these two ways of allocating funds. Those where patients follow funding promote cost control but narrow the choices of patients, and those where funding follows patients broaden the choices of patients but sacrifice some cost control. When efficiency means cost control, as it often does, it competes with choice.

Britain and New Zealand have experimented extensively with internal public markets in health care in the past decade. In the expectation that efficiency would improve, they moved to a model where patients follow funding. What does the evidence tell us? The promise of efficiency, it turns out, is much greater than the realization. Competition did not develop in public markets in either country, and when it did, few of the expected efficiencies materialized. For defenders of markets, the story is largely disappointing.

In one kind of public market, governments step back from direct management and create, at least in theory, an arm's-length authority, giving it full control of the budget. These health authorities, as they are generally called, assess the needs of their population across the health-care spectrum — not only for acute care, but for primary care as well; not only for medical care, but also for health care; and not only for treatment, but for prevention. They then go into the market and contract providers to meet the needs they have identified. Health authorities, the argument goes, can then reward efficient providers. These kinds of financial arrangements with health authorities at the centre have been established in Great Britain and New Zealand — both public systems that universalize care.[65] Their experience tells us that competition, the critical mechanism of efficiency, failed to develop in the way the architects of reform had hoped.

A second kind of public market, compatible with the first and, indeed, part of the British public market, requires that general practitioners become fundholders or purchasers of services for their patients. The concept relies on market dynamics within the framework of the public purse. Patients choose only their primary-care physician, who then acts as their agent to buy the care they need. In the United Kingdom, patients now follow the money; they no longer have the choice to leave their primary-care group.[66] Ironically, this public market narrowed individual choice to promote efficiency. That is not how it is supposed to work.

These group practices of family physicians are given a budget from the local health authority to buy care for their patients — elective hospital services, specialist services, diagnostic services, and prescription medicines. This kind of market makes physicians financially responsible for the care they prescribe.[67] Global budgets for doctors and competition for patients would create efficiencies in the critical part of the medical-care system that, some allege, drives costs.

How has it worked? How have arguments come to life? More than ten years of experience with public markets in Britain tells a cautionary tale. Fundholders did hold down the costs of prescription drugs in the first few years after they were created, but they did so largely by using generic alternatives rather than by reducing the number of prescriptions. After the first few years, however, cost reductions levelled off.[68] Another "efficiency" that was anticipated was a reduction in referrals to specialists. Here, too, the evidence is at best inconclusive.[69]

A second fundamental element of market logic was also muted. Competition — the quintessential hallmark of a market — was now explicitly discouraged in favour of cooperation between purchasers and providers. Competition, in order to work its magic, requires some excess capacity in the system that can be eliminated. But it proved no easier in a public market to close a local hospital than it has in Canada. Even more important, those who were buying care found that they had to cooperate with those who could provide the care. Most of the market incentives have been gradually removed from the British public market.[70]

The experiment in public markets in Britain — with government-appointed purchasers buying care in the market and general practitioners buying care on behalf of their patients — did not accomplish what was expected. Markets, in theory, provide efficiency through competition and the capacity to shut down those that are inefficient. This is not what happened; competition among purchasers is virtually non-existent, and competition among providers is very limited. In March 2000, the Labour government announced new funding of £19.4 billion for the National Health System, which, Tony Blair lamented, still "needs fundamental reform."[71]

How would this kind of system work in Canada? Public markets of regional health authorities that fully control their budgets and groups of primary-care physicians who buy care for their patients would narrow patient choice. Patients would still be able to choose, but only within their group of primary-care physicians. The critical question then becomes: How much choice — and what kind — do Canadians want? And how much freedom of choice would we give up in return for very modest gains in efficiency? The argument is turned on its head: public markets in publicly funded systems do not deliver efficiency *and* choice, but efficiency (in theory, if not in practice) *or* choice.

A "Smarter" State: The Arrow to Accountability

Public markets, like their private counterparts, do not eliminate the need for government — they change what governments do. Government is still present, but in a different way. It is no longer a hands-on manager, but rather a regulator, monitor, and evaluator of the way public goods are delivered and the way resources are allocated. Above all, government is the guardian of the public interest.[72] What governments do may be more costly in public markets than what they do as managers. The information they require to create and regulate public markets in health care and education is considerable: they have to provide "consumer" protection when they contract for services, certify providers, and extensively monitor and evaluate results. All of these require active — and often expensive — government action. At the very least, the costs of new and potentially large amounts of information are added to the government side of the ledger. Although the costs are real, the great benefit of public markets may well be, ironically, a smarter state.

The new smarter state will demand accountability from its public partners, who must in turn be accountable to each other and to the public. It is consequently no surprise that political voices from left to right are insisting on greater accountability. The demand for accountability crosses ideological lines. Markets assume accountability, the smart state needs accountability, and we as citizens have a right to accountability. To make meaningful judgements about efficiency, we need good assessments of effectiveness, and good assessments of effectiveness are the critical prerequisite to holding providers of public goods accountable.

The future of public goods will be fought on the battlefield of the standards of effectiveness that accountability requires. Constructing accountability is, in practice, not easy. Standards of performance are fundamentally contested, and choosing measures is a deeply political process, embedded in institutional legacies, cultural traditions, and social structures. We talk about the challenges of accountability in the next chapter.

Choice, Not Efficiency

I argued earlier that neither markets nor states offer ideal solutions to the delivery of public goods. Rather, each has its advantages and each creates its own kind of inefficiencies. Looking beyond the arguments to lived experience shows us that in health care, allowing public funds to flow to private institutions outside a framework of universal access does not provide clear advantages in cost-effectiveness and it is not efficient at maintaining equity. Genuinely public markets do not compromise equity, but they bring few significant gains in cost-effectiveness. And when they seek to control costs, they constrain choice. Neither do they deliver significant gains in efficiency, even when they limit choice.

In education, the story is a little different. Neither public funding of private institutions nor public markets increase efficiency, but they do increase choice. When public funding of private schools is restricted, it does increase equity. So do public markets. This is no small irony, given the often fiercely partisan lines of debate that argue the reverse. When Arthur Levine, the president of Columbia University Teachers' College, grew frustrated by the failure to improve inner-city schools, he called for a voucher plan for two to three million children at the worst urban schools. "For me," Levine said, "it's the equivalent of Schindler's list."[73] Public markets — charter schools — also empower and satisfy parents and build community. Markets in education and health care do not deliver what they promise — efficiency — but, at least in education, they provide what was not expected — choice, the strengthening of local community, and under certain conditions, greater equity.

The rhetoric of efficiency is deceptive. Given the record so far, the passionate support for public markets that we hear in public conversations cannot be about efficiency. If public markets do not deliver the efficiencies they promise, how then are we to understand the continuing fascination with the language of markets in public life? It is, as the king of Siam said in *The King and I,* a puzzlement.

Support for choice within public education is real and growing.[74] When the Children's Scholarship Fund in the United States offered 40,000 scholarships, or vouchers, to children from low-income families last year, more than 1.25 million applied. Support for charters and for choice within the public system could be understood as an escape from the weight of educational bureaucracies and government management, but government remains very much present, only in new ways. School choice does not rid citizen-consumers of government; on the contrary, consumers of education are simultaneously citizens who urgently need government to provide information about equality so that they can make informed choices.

Beneath the surface of the conversation about efficiency is a deeper debate about the intrinsic value of choice. Choice has become a value and is increasingly construed as a right. Indeed, support for choice long predates the current preoccupation with vouchers and charters. It began in the 1960s in Canada as an attempt to provide alternative schools for children and families who sought greater child-centred education than the public school system could provide. The debate about Ontario's controversial tax-credit program, which financially assists parents who send their children to private schools, is also about choice. "It's about recognizing that there are different philosophies and religious points of view," explains one parent, "and that we, as parents, need to have choice in education for our children."[75]

Parents do report far greater satisfaction when they

choose the school that their child attends, despite the limited progress, if any, that their children make in
improving their knowledge and skills. The metaphor of
choice carries value independent of evidence.[76] Parents
are more satisfied both because they have chosen their
child's school and because the act of choosing often leads
to greater engagement with the school and with other
parents who have made the same choice. The debate
about efficiency, when we dig beneath the surface, turns
very little on means and very much on the deeper values
of individual choice and community — and on their very
real consequences for equity and civic democracy.

Choice is challenging — and demanding. Parents
need to do research and assess the information they
receive. While filling out forms at an information session
about which public school they preferred for their children, one parent wistfully lamented, "I think all schools
should be equal. Then you wouldn't have to pick."[77]
Another parent celebrated the opportunity to choose and
the way it empowered her child and her family.

Some of the same dynamics are at work in health care
as well. If parallel private systems are not demonstrably
more cost-effective than public systems and are clearly
more inefficient at being equitable, why then the growing
public conversation around private alternatives to the
publicly funded medical-care system? David Gratzer, one
of the most vocal critics of medicare, is explicit:

> A commonly voiced argument in favour of the concept [of
> two-tier medicine] — one that is perhaps closest to the

hearts of the proponents of the private option — *has nothing to do with practical implications.* Proponents wonder why the state infringes on the liberties of citizens when it comes to health care. In our society, it is commonly accepted that citizens have the right to spend their money basically as they please.[78]

The underlying issue, Gratzer makes clear, is not efficiency, but choice.

Much of the current conversation about health care and public education is best understood as a conversation not only about efficiency — however it is defined — but, even more so, about choice and its limits. Beneath the cult of efficiency is a growing culture of choice. The right to choice, and the empowerment it brings, is the central instrument of a democratic society. It is no surprise that this debate is spilling over from our formal political institutions — and from the private marketplace — into our conversation about public goods.

IV

MEASURING UP:
CONSTRUCTING
ACCOUNTABILITY

*Here you can go into McDonald's and have a reasonable assur
ance that the french fries and the Big Mac will taste the same
whether you're in a small centre or a big centre. Of course, providing high-quality health care is a shade more complex than
making hamburgers and french fries! But when you consider
how much more important it is to have high-quality care for
patients, it's really hard to understand why we don't have the
same systematic approach to standard-setting and auditing to
ensure the quality of the health-care system.*

— David Naylor[1]

*I think it's reasonable for the public to say, "We want to know
how our schools are doing." But unless educators build up their
ability to work with testing, it's going to be a blunt instrument.*
— Michael Fullan[2]

FOUR YEARS AGO in Toronto, a newborn infant, Jordan
Heikamp, living with his teenage mother in a shelter run

by the Catholic Children's Aid Society, died of starvation. None of the trained social workers who saw him noticed that the baby was slowly starving to death. No criminal charges were laid after the baby died, but a coroner's inquest was held. The inquest concluded that the death was a homicide, but that the young mother was not completely responsible. Not one of the many social workers who testified accepted responsibility for the death of the child. The head of the Catholic Children's Aid Society was relieved by the verdict because, she said, Jordan's death was clearly a "systems failure."

"Everyone is nicely off the hook," observed the journalist Margaret Wente.

> Their motto might as well have been "No blame, no shame.". . . To hear the parade of social workers and their bosses tell it, they were victims too. . . . We never heard the word "accountability." Not one worker involved with Jordan was ever disciplined. . . . No jobs were lost, no operations shut down, no funding withdrawn. . . . Jordan died of chronic starvation. And of the culture of cruelly low expectations.[3]

Although a homicide had occurred, it was "the system" that had failed. No one within that system was held accountable. The coroner's jury made recommendations, lessons were learned, but throughout it all, there was no accountability. Wente was not the only one to understand that something was terribly wrong. Intuitively, people sensed that the absence of accountability, the failure to accept responsibility, is corrosive of private life and public institutions.

Public accountability is a fundamental right of citizens in a democratic polity. Without accountability, democracy does not work: there is no constraint on the arbitrary exercise of authority. But accountability is difficult to construct and enforce, even in democratic systems of responsible government. Accountability is even more challenging when states turn to markets for public goods, when the powers of the state are delegated and authority is one step or more further removed. What accountability means, how it is constructed, and what measures are important are part of a much larger conversation about values and purposes. To ignore accountability, or to dismiss it as a technical problem best left to the experts, is to miss one of the most important conversations of post-industrial society.

Public Accountability in the Post-industrial Age

Accountability is not difficult in an ideal, perfectly competitive private market. Unless firms collude, which they more than occasionally do, or selectively conceal information, which more than occasionally happens, the mechanisms of the market weed out the inefficient. Accountability in the marketplace is enforced through failure.

Private markets, however, do not provide public accountability. They do not build on the same concept of accountability that citizens — and now states — expect. Markets need to know only whether firms are profitable, not whether the goods and services that firms supply are as effective as they can be for the cost. Individual firms *do* care about effectiveness. They need to satisfy their customers or they will go out of business, so they are constantly trying to improve the quality and value of the goods and services they sell. The challenge is to improve quality while still remaining profitable.

This is the model of accountability that advocates bring with them when they propose public markets for public goods. But public accountability is more demanding. Citizens have the right to hold their leaders accountable for enforcing the laws they are sworn to uphold, for respecting the rights of citizens, and for acting in the public, rather than in their private, interest. There lies the critical difference. The less cynical would add that leaders are accountable for fulfilling the commitments they have made to the public and, more broadly, for fulfilling the will of the people.

Citizens have the right to know about the performance of leaders and institutions, and the right to judge that performance against consensually agreed upon standards. When performance falls short of these standards, citizens expect responsibility and responsiveness. Accountability means little if there are no consequences for those who fail to meet the standards, if problems are not addressed, if performance does not improve. And, in a democracy, if leaders do not respond to demands for accountability, citizens can reject them at the ballot box the next time they vote.

In ancient Athens, citizens were easily able to hold

leaders accountable because they participated directly in public decision making. Officials were directly accountable to citizens of the Assembly: there was extensive open debate, decisions were made after lengthy discussion, and there were consequences for failure to meet standards.[4] The Greek historian Xenophon tells of a great naval victory in 406 BC; many sailors died and those in command were accused of leaving men in wrecked boats to drown. "Back home," Xenophon wrote, "the People removed from office all the Generals except Konon. . . . Afterwards, there was a meeting of the Assembly, at which a number of people . . . attacked the Generals, saying that they should be called upon to explain why they had not rescued the men who had been shipwrecked."[5]

Athenians could hold their leaders accountable because those who were eligible for citizenship — not women or slaves, mind you — could come together directly in the *polis*, and engage in face-to-face public conversation, and if necessary, sanction their leaders. Athenians gave to subsequent generations the ideal of public accountability and its essential mechanisms. The ideal, but not the Athenian practice, remains with us.

As populations grew and political systems became more complex, democratic theory and practice had to change. As citizenship and the right to vote were gradually extended, publics became too large and too far-flung to come together and participate directly in public conversation. From this dilemma grew the ingenious invention of representative democracy. People elected representatives to express their will, and these representatives came together in parliaments. The accountability of government to its citizens was now one step removed, indirect rather than direct: the government would be accountable to parliament and parliament would be accountable to citizens.

In representative democracies, it is more difficult for citizens to hold governments accountable, because elected representatives act on behalf of their constituents. They become, in contemporary language, our agents. Agents often have interests of their own in addition to the interests of those "principals" they represent. If I wanted to sell our home, for example, I would hire a real-estate agent to act on my behalf. The relationship between the agent and the principal — in this case, me, the homeowner — seems fairly uncomplicated. There is more here, however, than meets the eye. The agent would want to sell the house as quickly as possible so that she could earn a commission, and she might encourage me to lower the price so that a sale could go through. Is the agent acting wholly in my interest or partly in her own? When the agent's interests do not coincide perfectly with those of the principal, and they almost never do, problems can develop. These problems are relatively simple in the relationship between a real-estate agent and a homeowner, but they are far more complex and multi-dimensional in public life, where voters have multiple interests and their elected representatives have the interests of their political party and their own careers to consider, as well as their responsibility to the voters. It is these "principal-agent dilemmas" that create some of the biggest challenges to the exercise of political accountability in public life.[6]

One solution to principal-agent dilemmas in public life is to limit the scope of political accountability. Max Weber had a narrow vision of accountability that contrasted dramatically with the practice in ancient Athens. Weber explained that the "emotionality" of the masses made them incapable of judging public issues and urged that the role of voters be limited to choosing able leaders and dismissing the incompetent.[7] Citizens were therefore to be empowered only at the beginning and end of the electoral cycle. The classical liberal democratic tradition upon which Weber built consistently tried both to defend and to limit accountability to citizens.[8] As industrialization accelerated, this highly restrictive concept of accountability was a comfortable fit with the hierarchical, command-and-control bureaucratic state that was developing.

However, the very limited accountability of their leaders began to sit far less comfortably with citizens as the social welfare state grew and reached more and more deeply into people's lives. The demand for broader accountability increased, but there were formidable challenges. We have already examined the challenges that principal-agent dilemmas create. Add to these the problems that contemporary democracies pose for the exercise of accountability. In our parliamentary democracy, when we vote every four years or so, issues are bundled together; we have to vote for our representatives, and their parties, on a take-it-or-leave-it basis. Accountability for specific issues on a day-to-day basis is clouded by our system of cyclical elections. Party discipline and Cabinet government further stifle the capacity to hold officials accountable. Not even parliamentarians are truly Athenian citizens any longer; free votes — where representatives are allowed to vote on an issue as their conscience dictates, rather than as party policy mandates — are rare in our parliamentary system. Moreover, the hierarchical bureaucratic state was reluctant to release information about performance, and to evaluate openly the effectiveness of the public goods it delivered. These structural problems led to a growing "democratic deficit," and fed public scepticism about political leaders and public institutions.

In his 1965 Massey Lectures, the political theorist C. B. Macpherson argued passionately that even in densely populated, complex democracies, participation and accountability can be extended. Voting in elections once every four or five years is not enough. Citizens cannot be involved in face-to-face discussions every time a public issue that is important to them is on the agenda, nor would they want to be. But, Macpherson argued, political parties can be reorganized to become less hierarchical, and they can be made more accountable and responsive to their local constituencies. Political parties could also be constrained through greater democracy in the workplace and in the community, where face-to-face discussion is eminently feasible and direct accountability is possible. Macpherson called this process participatory democracy.[9] With participation would come accountability.

Participatory democracy — and with it, the opportunity for broader and deeper accountability — is extraordinarily difficult to implement. National arenas, with large populations and a multiplicity of issues, are not a fair test of Macpherson's ideas. Not only is geographical space too broad, but the scope of the "political" — the formal institutions of government and the political parties that work within them — may be too narrow. As the reach of the state has grown, the "political" encompasses far more: the whole set of institutions, policies, and players — both private and public — that provide public goods that are fundamental to citizens.

We, as citizens of the post-industrial state, understand the changing political terrain. We do not feel heard by our elected representatives, but we are increasingly willing to engage in unconventional political participation on issues that matter to us. Public education and health care directly touch all of us sooner or later; we feel that we do have the capacity to make judgements about these issues, even when they are complex. We are more and more inclined to demand clearer standards of performance, better information, and greater responsiveness from leaders and officials. And as the culture of choice deepens in the post-industrial age, we are demanding greater accountability from our representatives, who are our agents, so that we can make better decisions as citizens.

It is not only citizens who are demanding greater accountability. The new smarter state, as we saw in the previous chapter, is becoming the buyer of public goods on our behalf, rather than the direct provider, as it was during the industrial age. The state is becoming the buyer because it seeks to improve efficiency in the way public goods are provided. The state as buyer requires accountability as it backs out of the delivery of public goods, devolves authority down, and contracts out service delivery.

When the state directly delivered and managed public goods — when it rowed the boat — it had little incentive to be transparent and accountable. Accountability would subject its performance to critical review and reveal its mistakes. The annual release of the auditor general's report still strikes terror in the hearts of senior civil servants. Now that the state is buying services — from schools it charters, from clinics it funds — now that it is experimenting with public markets and steering rather than rowing, it has every reason to demand accountability.[10]

There is real irony here. The state changed its shape to improve efficiency — a promise that, as we have seen, has not materialized — but the permanent legacy may well be a much richer agenda of accountability. When efficiency is used to mean cost-effectiveness, knowledge of what is and is not effective becomes essential. This is exactly the knowledge that states need from those who provide public goods, and that citizens need in order to hold their institutions accountable. The state and the citizen are allies — at times uneasy allies — in demanding accountability from those who provide public goods. The language of efficiency in public life carries with it the seeds of a more important vocabulary of accountability.

If we as citizens cannot imagine how we can hold our

local schools and hospitals accountable, then it is far less likely that we can imagine how we can hold the educational and health-care systems, much less our governments, accountable. Even holding a local school accountable, however, is more complicated than it seems at first glance. We first ask, What does accountability mean? How is its meaning constructed? And then, Accountable for what? Accountable how? Accountable to whom? We begin the discussion of accountability in the larger arena of public life with a discussion of how meaningful accountability might be achieved in the smaller arena of health care and education.

Building in Accountability

There are those who root the fundamental problems of accountability in education and health care in the institutions that govern the systems — the school boards, hospital boards, ministries, and governments — and in the incentives they create for educators and providers of health care. Developing explicit standards of performance, drawing up a charter of rights for parents and patients, carefully evaluating effectiveness — these are all system-preserving reforms that tinker at the edges. Accountability for performance, the argument goes, can be had only by changing the rules of the system.

Proponents of school choice through public markets argue that only by meeting the demands of parents who are free to change schools — to "exit" if they are dissatisfied — will accountability improve. Public markets are created when the state takes a step back and uses public money to contract others — public institutions, private and not-for-profit organizations — to provide our most important public goods. In a public market, the state funds providers, monitors performance, and makes sure that schools disclose full information to parents so that they can make the best choices. The argument is that accountability will come from a radical change in structure and incentives, not from the development of yet another process, yet another standard, yet another test, yet another code of conduct, and yet one more area of bureaucratic management and control. Push responsibility down and free parents to choose; create a public market, and accountability will follow naturally from competition.

Advocates of public markets in health care make parallel, though less extensive, claims. The argument in health care is similar to the reasoning in education but more complicated, because the delivery of health care includes so many overlapping layers of delegation. Governments are accountable to their citizens; those who buy health care on behalf of governments are accountable to citizens and to the government; and those who provide health care are accountable to those who buy it, as well as to their patients. There are difficult principal-agent dilemmas in each of these relationships, and they are made worse because both purchasers and providers of health care in public markets are accountable to more than one principal.[11] To give citizens the most cost-effective health care, the challenge is to balance the political and financial incentives of the state, of the purchasers who act on its behalf, and of providers of care. This is no easy task.

Public markets, their defenders claim, can help. Competition will work its magic, advocates of public markets suggest, providing not only greater efficiency but also better accountability, if we can get the political and financial incentives right. Accountability, they say, grows out of competition.[12]

How do these arguments live with the experience in public markets of the past decade? The record in education and health care does not suggest that accountability improved markedly when public markets were introduced. To be fair, the argument has never been fully tested because competition did not develop in the United Kingdom and New Zealand, the two great laboratories of public health-care markets. Without competition, the dynamic of accountability that advocates of public markets expect never had a chance to work.

But it is no accident that competition did not flourish as expected. Governments were reluctant to dismantle many of the regulations they had put in place to keep costs under control. When efficiency is a cult among political leaders, when cost-containment and cost-cutting are political ends, it constrains the way public markets work. This is not what advocates of public markets expected. More to the point, health-care buyers and providers need to cooperate with one another as much as they need to compete. Competition, the bedrock of the argument for public markets, can take us only so far.

In public education, the story is different. When structures were changed and public markets were created

through school choice, charter schools were often not subject to the same rigorous standards of evaluation as
schools within the regular public system.[13] Ironically, the
public market in education has created a two-tier system
of accountability.

The problem goes even deeper. Even if competition
could be heightened in public health-care markets, and
even if all schools in the public system were tested in
exactly the same way, citizens would still need to know
what health-care providers and educators are accountable for. What is it that we expect from those who buy
health care on our behalf, and from those who deliver it to
us? What is it that we expect from those who provide
education to our children? These are hard questions that
go to our basic values, values that touch on how we think
about ourselves and our societies. The *what* of accountability matters, and it is the first essential that must be in
place before we can even begin to talk about *how* we wish
to hold our governments, our buyers, and our providers
accountable in public markets.

What meaning has been given to accountability in
practice? How has it lived? In the United Kingdom and
New Zealand, governments, health-care purchasers,
and providers all agreed on "quality of care" as the goal.
Who would disagree? But if we look beneath the rhetoric, we see that quality was not measured at all in Britain
in the first wave of reforms in the 1980s and 1990s. Performance was measured by the volume and rate of
growth of "finished episodes" of care — how many
patients went through the system — a measure that

made no pretence of evaluating whether treatment was effective or appropriate![14] This kind of measure taps productive efficiency and would work as well in Adam Smith's pin factory. If quality of care is the goal of the health-care system but quality is neither measured nor evaluated, accountability, just like efficiency, remains at the level of rhetoric.

In the past five years, governments in New Zealand and the United Kingdom have done more. They publish annual guidelines establishing objectives and setting standards of performance for the purchasers of health care. The objectives are general, inclusive, and rhetorical: equity, effectiveness, efficiency, safety, and acceptability. Again, digging beneath the conversation to look at the practice, we see that monitoring has concentrated on a small number of highly visible issues: waiting times, annual activity, and the health of at-risk populations.[15] Not surprisingly, providers of health care focus their efforts on those standards that are monitored. Public markets in health are no different from public education, where standardized tests have set the bar and teachers teach to the test. What is measured matters, because what is measured is what people do.

Measuring Up: The Construction of Accountability

Measures of effectiveness — the political terrain on which the battles of accountability are fought — are constructed in society. What is considered effective in one historical period is judged ineffective — and at times unacceptable — in another. Take, for example, corporal punishment as an instrument of effective education. Until quite recently, schools across Canada were free to use corporal punishment to instil discipline in the classroom. Few questioned or tested its effectiveness. Today, very few schools would defend the use of physical punishment, even if it were demonstrably effective as a motivator of learning. I suspect that the change is not a result of rigorously controlled studies documenting that the use of the strap lowers test scores. Far more likely, changing values in an altered social environment made the use of physical punishment unacceptable. And so it is with almost all measures and evaluations of educational and health-care strategies. Our choice of measures and the meanings we attribute to standards engage our most basic values and purposes.

It matters profoundly which measures of effectiveness are chosen. It matters because these measures — once they are socially accepted — feed back to, and drive, the performance of those who provide public goods. Schools and hospitals began only recently, for example, to measure parent and patient satisfaction. To some, this is a frivolous, fuzzy measure. What does it matter whether parents and patients are satisfied? What is important is that students learn what they need to know, and that patients receive cost-effective treatment. However, we do know that a sense of efficacy does matter: patients who are empowered tend to follow their course of treatment more carefully and recover more quickly, and parents who are satisfied are more likely to become involved in their children's homework and school. So customer service and customer satisfaction can be related to better results in education and in health care. Since satisfaction does contribute to better outcomes, including it as a measure of effectiveness is an easy decision.

Imagine for a moment that parent and patient satisfaction did not contribute to better outcomes. Would it still make sense to include them as measures of effectiveness? Some would argue that fiscally constrained education and health-care systems cannot afford to concentrate on anything that does not clearly improve outcomes. Others, myself included, would argue that the fundamental right of every person to dignity and respect makes parent and patient satisfaction a valuable measure, independent of its impact on outcomes. When we ask to whom our local public school and community hospital is accountable, the answer must be, in part, to parents and patients. This answer is driven by values. The local public school and community hospital are also part of larger systems of public education and public health care, which are ultimately accountable to the public. The choice of what to measure then becomes a public issue, and this choice is only partly a matter of technical expertise. Far more often, it is a matter of values.

If accountability is to have teeth, the measures of effectiveness have to be reported in ways that we as citizens can understand. It is through this process of transparent public reporting that a chain of accountability is created in a mature democratic society. Weber's distrust of the public, a distrust that he expressed a century ago, jars with our post-industrial sensibility that we are capable of understanding complex issues and coming to judgement. The language of accountability in a democracy is devoid of meaning — it is a conceit and a deceit — if the institutions that provide our public goods do not report what they do and how well they accomplish the charge we have given them.

Measuring Educational Success

Accountability in public education is multi-layered. The system of public education is accountable to society as a whole; schools are accountable to parents, students, and boards; boards are accountable to the government; teachers are accountable to the school, parents, students, and their professional associations; and students are accountable to teachers, parents, and fellow students. Let us turn our attention to only one piece of this big jigsaw puzzle — the accountability of schools within the system of public education. It can serve as a metaphor for the much larger question of the accountability of those who provide fundamental public goods.

The first difficult question is, Accountability for what? One of the leading voices for the voucher movement in the United States, Terry Moe, argues that what matters is that parents are happy. "Tens of thousands of parents," he concluded, "can't be wrong!"[16] The most important indicator of effectiveness becomes parent satisfaction. Here is one social construction of accountability rooted in the concept of citizen-consumer in the public market.

Modern followers of Jeremy Bentham and the utilitarians — the vanguard of the movement for efficiency —

would have no choice but to agree.[17] The standards are internal. If parents are satisfied, the school is succeeding. "Choice shifts accountability away from the government," Moe insists, "and towards the parent and the institutions that their children attend." When the argument is made this way, the problem with internal standards as the only markers of effectiveness is laid bare. This is an exclusively market-based conception of accountability, where what matters is the satisfaction of the individual consumer. I suspect that few parents, and fewer citizens whose tax dollars are funding voucher students, would agree. Most would expect schools to be held accountable for more than the satisfaction of parents. They would expect student achievement to improve over time.

There is widespread agreement that basic numeracy and literacy are fundamental requirements of any successful educational system. This is a second, quite different, construction of accountability that is rooted in the larger argument about what productive members of a post-industrial, knowledge-based economy will need. The most important determinant of the global location of production is the quality of the workforce. A better-educated workforce is the best investment post-industrial societies could make to enhance their capacity to compete in a knowledge-intensive global economy. "Education has long been recognized as an important contributor to economic growth," argued George Radwanski, the author of an influential report to the Ontario Ministry of Education in 1988, "but now it has become *the* paramount ingredient for competitive success in the world economy."[18] Education has now regained the central role as an engine of growth that it had in the early and middle phases of industrialization.

This emphasis on education as the engine of the post-industrial economy has revolutionized the debate about education as a public good, and it has led directly to an emphasis on testing what students know and how they perform in comparison with their peers. Standardized testing of students swept through the educational world in the past decade. More than half a million students from fourth to twelfth grade in forty-one countries have participated in three rounds of testing in science and mathematics.[19] Are you interested in how Canada scored? If you are, you have just instinctively given some weight to standardized testing as a measure of the effectiveness of public education that is rooted largely in the requirements of the post-industrial economy. Canadian students in twelfth grade ranked tenth, behind students in the Netherlands, Sweden, and Iceland, but above the United States. The next question is, Are the results good enough? How do we judge?

For many, the results were judged not good enough. Governments — and parents — have agreed that basic literacy and numeracy is fundamental. The United States, the United Kingdom, and New Zealand, as well as Canada, have moved to state-led accountability of the public school system through standardized testing. In Canada, a nationally agreed upon project reports on the average ranking of participating provinces.[20] Some of the provinces have gone even further.[21] Responsibility for deciding whether or not a student graduates is no longer simply that of the local school; it is now shared with the government. Beginning in 2002, secondary-school students in Ontario who fail the compulsory literacy test will not be allowed to graduate.

The commitment of parents and citizens to the goal of basic literacy will be tested by fire when, for the first time, a significant group of students will be unable to graduate if they cannot pass a standardized test. Is this an appropriate price that we as citizen-consumers are willing to pay? The answer to that question — an important collective, as well as individual, decision   will come not only from parents, or even from citizens, but from governments that are now leading the drive for accountability. This is the new regulating and monitoring state: it is setting standards and assuring quality based on its construction of what students need in the post-industrial age.

It is no surprise that standardized testing has provoked fierce controversy and protest from parents and teachers who reject a unidimensional measure of knowledge. The tests are fast, easy, and relatively inexpensive to administer; scored by machines, they are far less expensive to grade than essay questions. "Efficient tests," argued one specialist, "tend to drive out less efficient tests, leaving many important abilities untested — and untaught."[22] The cost side of the equation is clear, but the effectiveness is not." As the mechanical facilities of our educational institutions expand," writes Lewis Mumford in his brilliant analysis of the impact of automation on

society, "with their heavy investment in . . . their comput-
ers . . . their machine-marked 'yes-or-no' examination
papers, the human content necessarily shrinks in significance. . . . The constant dialogue that is so necessary for
self-knowledge, for social cooperation, and for moral
evaluation and rectification, has no place in an automated
regimen."[23]

Criticism of standardized testing comes in many
colours and shapes. At issue is what the tests test, how the
results are used, and whom the tests hurt and help. The
debate is particularly intense precisely because the test
results inform judgements of accountability as well as
effectiveness: it is not only students' careers that are on
the line, but the future of teachers and principals. It is no
surprise, by the way, that the incidence of cheating has
risen dramatically as the use of high-stakes tests has
increased.[24] Testing has changed the incentives of students, teachers, principals, and school boards, as well as
governments.

The "what" of accountability is fiercely contested. The
basic issue is the kind of knowledge that is being measured. Some educators accept the need for scientific and
mathematical thinking in a knowledge-based economy,
but they argue that standardized tests measure the wrong
kind of knowledge. Multiple-choice tests that can most
easily be scored emphasize memorization, recognition,
technical skills, and the capacity to find quick answers
rather than to reflect. These kinds of tests, attractive
because they are so easy to use, do tell us something, but
only about a certain kind of limited knowledge. "These

tests," wrote Howard Gardner of the Harvard Graduate School of Education, "don't measure whether students can think scientifically or mathematically, they just measure a kind of lowest common denominator of facts and skills. So getting students to do well on them doesn't mean much in the real world."[25]

Others go much further and deeper. Richard Atkinson, the president of the University of California, the largest and one of the most prestigious public systems of higher education in the United States, sent shock waves through the educational community recently. Echoing Lewis Mumford, he recommended that the University of California no longer make the standardized aptitude test (known universally as the SAT) a requirement of admission. He urged its nine campuses to move away from admission processes that use quantitative formulas, and instead look at prospective students "in a comprehensive, holistic way."[26] This kind of admission procedure, Atkinson argued, would free high schools from their current preoccupation with test-taking skills rather than education.

Atkinson could have turned to the philosopher John Dewey for support for an educational system that develops the full potential of each individual student. "A common error," Dewey argued, "is the assumption that there is one set body of subject matter and skills to be presented to the young, only requiring to be presented and 'learned' by the child, whose failure to meet the material supplied is attributed to his own incapacity or willfulness, not to failure of the educator to understand what needs are stirring him."[27] The public philosopher John Ralston Saul, like the ancient Greeks before him, articulated a second vision in his 1995 Massey Lectures: "The existence of a high-quality national education system for the first dozen years or so of training is the key to a democracy where legitimacy lies with the citizen."[28] Here the critique goes deeper — to the individual potential and diverse strengths of each student, and to the broader academic and civic purposes of education that standardized aptitude tests cannot capture.

Critics go beyond the kind of knowledge — and education — that tests reward and ask whom these tests hurt. Standardized tests, they allege, systematically favour students from a homogeneous cultural and socio-economic background — the white middle class. Students who come from low-income families, and who do not quickly grasp school culture and the dominant mode of teaching and learning, will not do well on these kinds of tests.[29] The uniformity and apparent equity of tests contributes to real-world inequity — through lowered expectations and tracking. Critics charge that standardized testing is a pernicious kind of accountability to those students in public schools who need the most help.

Advocates of testing disagree strongly. They insist that literacy and numeracy are the essential prerequisites of innovation and critical thinking, of educated citizens, and of a fulfilled individual. This is a compelling argument. Michael Fullan, a pioneer in educational reform, agrees that testing based on clear — and comparative — standards of literacy and numeracy is an important measure of effectiveness. "In the age of accountability," he concludes, "testing is not going away."[30] Where students are deficient, practice and reinforcement of basic literacy and numeracy skills is precisely what schools need to do to improve achievement. Testing, Fullan argues, can provide the necessary leverage, the shock, to cut through bureaucracy and spur improvement.[31] If governments focus only on the accountability of the schools, Fullan adds, they will do more harm than good.[32] How test results are used also matters. If schools are held accountable by governments for doing better than expected, then governments must be held accountable to help those schools that are not performing well. Accountability is reciprocal and mutually obligating.

Finally, there is the "how" of accountability. The way the results of standardized tests are presented often compromises accountability. Test results are often used to rank some students, schools, or provinces, as above average and others as below average.[33] Some standardized tests do measure a student's level of knowledge — the Ontario literacy test is a good example — but most are focused not so much on what students know, but on how they compare with every other student taking the test. Tests deliberately include extraordinarily difficult questions so that some students will be at the top, most will bunch in the middle, and some will be at the bottom.

Using averages to measure educational performance is a curiously competitive standard. It tells us little about what students actually know, about how proficient they are, and instead assesses only whether they are better or worse than the average. In this kind of reporting, some students, schools, and provinces will always be below average, regardless of what the students know. This, after all, is the meaning of an average: some will always be above and some will always be below. However, this kind of reporting makes it appear that some students, or schools, or provinces, or countries, are doing terribly, no matter their level of proficiency. It creates the impression that some schools are failing, but by the way the results are presented, some schools must always fail. When we ask how schools are held accountable, the answer must be that the way some results are presented builds in failure.

The *Report Card*, issued by the Fraser Institute, is a good example of how not to use comparative measures to judge effectiveness.[34] The report uses five measures of academic achievement, aggregates the measures, and ranks all schools across a province. It does compensate for socio-economic status in its published rankings, but it ranks private schools in the same pool with public schools. Since the socio-economic status of students is derived from data supplied by provincial ministries, information for private-school students is not as readily available or reliable. It is not unreasonable to assume that students in private schools generally come from higher-than-average-income families, with better-educated parents. Private schools are also free, of course, to reject students. The *Report Card* in 2001 produced no surprises: private schools led the list of effective schools in Ontario. The result: the status of private schools is enhanced, and the public school system is degraded — owing to an unfair comparison. At the very least, private and public schools should be ranked in two separate pools. The "how" of accountability matters: the devil is truly in the details.

Even when the test tests what students know, the results are almost always presented in an across-the-board comparison. The percentage of students who passed the literacy test in each high school in Ontario was published in newspapers across the province. Parents eagerly scanned the paper for their child's school, comparing its percentage of passes with other schools. But this kind of presentation made no allowance for differences of socio-economic background by district, for the number of children for whom English was a second language, or for the number of students in special-education programs.

The principal of the high school that had the highest percentage of students who passed in Toronto was refreshingly honest. In Ashley Waltman's school, 91 percent of the students passed the test, compared with an average of 55 percent who passed in the Toronto District School Board and 61 percent who passed across the province. But Waltman warned against interpreting the results to mean that his school is more effective than others. Instead, he explained, the high pass rate largely reflects a student body free of the language and cultural barriers so many other schools face. "I really don't like all this comparison between schools," Waltman argued, "even though we're a beneficiary of it, because schools' results have so much to do with demographics. We have no program for English as a second language at our school and more than 90 percent of our students go on to university, so we have no demand for workplace-related courses. So with demographics like that you'd expect us to do well."[35]

Waltman is right. His school did only marginally better than would be expected when the socio-economic status of students is correlated with the results of the literacy tests. Doug Little, a former school trustee, was frustrated by the way the results of the Ontario literacy tests were published in newspapers across the province. He decided independently to match each school's success rate with the socio-economic background and special needs of its students. The results are striking: the lower the socio-economic background of a school and the needier its students, the lower the percentage of students who passed the test. "You could predict," explained Little, "that there would be a dramatic difference in literacy test scores based on class distinction."[36] The match was almost perfect — very few schools did significantly better, or worse, than expected. Kipling, a school where only 50 percent passed the literacy test, was one of the very few schools to do significantly better than expected. Given the socio-economic background of its students, it did much better than did Waltman's high-scoring school, which captured so much public attention. Little's presentation of results provides a meaningful measure of performance — and of accountability of teachers and principals.

No matter how intense the controversy, few would argue that schools should not be held accountable at all. Yet in private markets that are supported by public funds, the standards of state-led accountability are often less strict and at times entirely absent. The proposal by the government of Ontario to provide tax credits to students choosing private schools, as we saw in the previous chapter, runs a real risk of two-tier accountability. Public funds will be transferred to private schools that are not governed by provincial standards. Private schools in Ontario, if they receive no funding from the provincial government, do not have to administer the tests that are compulsory in the public primary-school system. Unless the government insists that parents who claim the tax credit restrict their choice to only those private schools that accept compulsory testing, it will have structured a blatant system of two-tier accountability; a double standard of accountability is transparently unjust.

Charter schools promise accountability largely through market failure, but in the United States, very few have been closed because they failed to meet academic standards. Closing schools that do not perform is the ultimate test of a public market, where schools are much less closely monitored and are free to deliver education as they see fit. Freedom from bureaucratic regulation is, after all, one of the principal advantages touted by proponents of public markets in education. It makes sense, however, only when it goes hand in hand with a willingness to close schools that are not performing. Otherwise, accountability through competition and choice will not work the way proponents of public markets expect.

If the market mechanism is not working, at the very least the same standards that apply to schools within the public system should apply to schools within the public market. Often they do not.[37] Standards of accountability vary widely — and wildly — in the public market of charter schools across the United States. Charter schools are less accountable than the increasingly regulated public school system. "Today's charter-school accountability systems remain underdeveloped," concludes one veteran observer, "often clumsy, and ill-fitting, and are themselves beset by dilemmas."[38] There is a growing system of two-tier accountability.

Critics disagree — often passionately — about what schools should be held accountable for, how they should be held accountable, and to whom they should be accountable. A revolt against standardized testing as the single measure of effectiveness and the only mechanism of accountability is growing. The tail of testing has begun to wag the educational dog. Parents are upset by the amount of classroom time taken from other teaching to prepare students to take the test. This wave of protest is led, not by the parents and teachers in schools whose students are performing poorly on standardized tests, but by schools in affluent neighbourhoods whose students generally do very well.[39]

The revolt against standardized testing goes deeper. It is partly a revolt against a construction of effectiveness that focuses too narrowly on the needs of the post-industrial economy; other kinds of skills — the capacity to think critically and to innovate — are just as important in the new knowledge economy, and standardized tests do not tap these kinds of abilities. It is partly a revolt against a construction of effectiveness that ignores the importance of public education to the creation of committed and engaged citizens. It is also a revolt against a construction of effectiveness that ignores the needs of the whole child.

Beneath the growing controversy surrounding testing as the principal mechanism of accountability lies a largely unheard conversation about the goals and values of public education. What are tests testing for? What are the values and purposes of public education? Good measures of effective public education are controversial and difficult to design. They are controversial because measures are constructed within our pictures of society, and these pictures differ. They are difficult because so many of us expect so much of our public schools: some want literate and numerate students; others give pride of place to critical and innovative thinkers; and others want all of that as well as knowledgeable, committed, and tolerant citizens. All of these are fair expectations of a system of public education.

Our expectations of our schools as parents, citizens, and a society are far too rich to be captured by a single test. The effectiveness — and accountability — of public schools cannot be assessed reliably by one measure alone. Reliance on quantitative measures, without the time-consuming qualitative judgements as an accompaniment, introduces significant bias into the assessment of accountability. It distorts what we teach, what our students learn, and even more, it disfigures the picture of our children, of education, and of our society. Choosing the most easily graded test — the efficient test — is a concept of efficiency that badly diminishes the educational system. If we try in the name of efficiency, or even of accountability, to use just a single measure, we create an impoverished set of incentives in our public system of education, a system that is the outward manifestation of our deepest dreams of citizenship and society. Our values and our common sense tell us that a broad array of qualitative and quantitative measures will better capture whether students have the kinds of knowledge they will need to be engaged and committed citizens, as well as productive members of society.

But most pernicious of all is to accept no accountability — creating, in Margaret Wente's words, "a culture of cruelly low expectations."[40] Students, parents, and citizens have a right to accountability — it is a defining attribute of democratic life. Negotiating the right mix of standards for an accountable public school system will define the debate about public education. Holding government accountable for helping schools that are ineffective will enrich public education and society. In the process, the smart state and engaged citizens become more important than ever.

Measuring Quality Care

Just as education is an outward manifestation of our deeper thinking about citizenship and society, so health care speaks to our most important collective values. Even more so than in education, governments, as we saw in the last chapter, have been experimenting with public markets to deliver health care more efficiently. As in education, the drive for efficiency in health care has created a new vocabulary of accountability. In health care, too, it is the "what" of accountability that is so difficult to construct and so contested.

The health-care system, paradoxically, cannot be held fully accountable for health. Health is no more a function of the health-care system than educational achievement is a product of the education system. If it were so, then how might we explain that with our seemingly problem-plagued health-care system, Canadians rank third in life expectancy, surpassed only by Iceland and Japan. Much of the credit for longer life expectancies actually belongs largely to improvements in income, diet, and sanitation. But the strongest determinant of life expectancy — and more broadly of health and educational success — is socio-economic status.[41] In Canada, and around the world, the poor are disproportionately sick.

Every hospital and every health-care system loudly proclaims as its most important objective the delivery of quality care. As part of every election campaign, political leaders recommit themselves to assuring and improving quality care. Political battles are fought on the terrain of quality care by physicians and other health-care professionals, who worry that intervention by the market or the state will jeopardize quality, and by political leaders and buyers of health care, who emphasize the need to enhance quality in the face of resistance by health-care professionals. But what does quality mean? How is it understood? How is it interpreted? How is it measured? Is the battle over quality a cover for other agendas?

I recently asked the head of a quality-assurance program in one of Canada's leading hospitals how he would want his hospital held accountable. After a moment of silence, he promised to write me a short note within a few days. "It troubles me at the outset," he wrote, "that I have no simple answer, particularly as the broad theme of 'accountability and performance measurement' has been a priority for our hospital in the past two years. My slight embarrassment over this matter has been cause for considerable introspection over the last few days. Should we even ask the question? I raise this question simply because I'm not yet convinced that judging hospitals or other providers of public services is even a useful exercise."[42] His hesitation is an honest reflection of the complexity of the task he faces.

The "to whom" as well as the "what" of accountability for quality is also contested. The same kinds of agency problems that bedevil public education make accountability in health care difficult. The health-care system as a whole is accountable to the public; health-care institutions — hospitals and clinics in the community, whether they are not-for-profit or private — are accountable to their patients, to their boards, and to the agencies and ministries that fund them; health-care professionals are accountable to their professional colleges, to their patients, and to the institutions in which they work; and patients are accountable for behaving sensibly and complying with the requirements of their treatments. Often, one agent — a doctor or a hospital — is accountable to several principals simultaneously. In a complex system of overlapping responsibilities, there is no simple answer to the question, Accountable to whom?

As we did when we looked at public education, we put only one node in the larger network — the hospital — under our microscope to shed light on broader patterns and problems of accountability within the larger health-care system. The hospital is becoming less and less significant in the overall health-care system, so it may seem a curious specimen to put under the microscope of accountability. I choose the hospital because it is where the vectors of government, professional, and public accountability converge.

For what have hospitals been held accountable in the name of quality? The word "quality" has come to have almost mystical significance. But in everyday language, we have a common-sense understanding that quality is connected to excellence. The construction of the meaning of quality in health care is far more modest. We generally understand quality as equitable and timely access to effective care. Do we get the care we need in a timely way, and is the care effective when we get it? Did our health-care provider do the right thing? How were we treated personally? All three dimensions — equitable access to timely care, the right care, and respectful care — together constitute quality and effectiveness.

Accountability in health care is given meaning by

those who buy it, by those who provide it, by consumers who need it now, and by all of us who know that we will need health care sometime in the future. Purchasers, providers, consumers, and society have different agendas, different goals, and at times, even different values. It is no surprise that they each want different standards of accountability for hospitals within the broader health-care system.

At least four groups of measures speak to these different agendas. We must start with effectiveness of treatment, for it is at the core of any concept of accountability. We cannot even begin to talk about the efficiency of health care unless we know first that it is effective. Satisfied patients who receive ineffective medical treatment would be as inappropriate a measure of a hospital as satisfied parents whose children remain unable to read would be an inappropriate measure of a school. Just as post-industrial society has determined that literacy and numeracy of students are the critical measures of the effectiveness of schools, so effectiveness of care is the critical measure of hospitals and doctors.

That agreement takes us only so far. As we just saw, the debate about what makes a school effective is boiling. There is a parallel debate about what constitutes effective care. More and more, in our knowledge-based society, we are turning to evidence. Evidence-based analysis of the outcomes and practice of health care speaks to everyone — the government that wants cost-effective care, health-care providers that set professional standards, patients who want the most effective treatment, and citizens who

expect state-of-the-art health care. Evidence-based practice is the first measure that we look at, but as we shall
see, the evidence does not speak for itself in health care
any more than it does in education.

A single concept of accountability did not work in
education and does not work in health care. Three other
measures also matter. Efficiency speaks loudly to governments, to those it appoints to buy health care, and to
citizens who want cost-effective care. Patient satisfaction
with the kind of care they receive, and particularly waiting lists and waiting times, speaks principally to citizen-
consumers. It is part of the larger agenda of citizens in a
post-industrial society, and it fits with our growing sense
of autonomy and empowerment. Finally, fair reporting
that is understandable to the public touches our deepest
values as citizens in a mature liberal democracy. None of
these four measures is easy to construct.

1) **Evidence-based outcomes and practice.** This group of
measures speaks to the capacity of the health-care professions to bring the best knowledge to bear on the care they
provide. "Did the procedure produce an improvement?"
asks Terry Sullivan, vice-president of Cancer Care
Ontario. "Did it make a difference?"[43] Measures of clinical
outcomes, just like the results of standardized tests, have
an intuitive appeal. The "best practices" that reflect the
most up-to-date knowledge should lead to the best outcomes.

It is surprising, even astounding to many of us, that
until a decade ago, most clinical practice was based

almost entirely on trial and error by experienced clini-
cians. Carefully controlled trials and systematic reviews
of evidence to establish the effectiveness of different treatments in producing better outcomes were rare. It was a
British medical researcher, Archie Cochrane, who, just
three decades ago, began to push relentlessly for more
evidence-based standards in the evaluation of the effectiveness of different treatments.[44] In 1993, medical experts
from nine countries first came together to found
the Cochrane Collaboration to review systematically the
effects of different medical interventions. Few patients
realize that systematic work on effectiveness is in its
infancy.

Just as measuring the effectiveness of education is
more complex than advocates of standardized testing
lead us to believe, so too is identification and measurement of clinical outcomes far more difficult than it
appears. Suppose our local hospital reported that one-
tenth of the patients who underwent bypass surgery for
coronary heart disease died within thirty days. How are
we to make sense of this result? Is such a death rate
higher than it should be? Lower? Is it a result of the care
the patients received while they were in the hospital? Did
this group of patients have particularly severe heart disease? Were they likely to have a higher-than-usual death
rate? What is usual? Unless we can answer these questions, we can make no sense at all of the information that
10 percent of the patients died within thirty days. We are
in no position to judge whether the hospital was performing adequately or failing.

What would we need to know to make sense of this information? The death rate begins to make some sort of sense only if we can compare mortality rates in other hospitals or the rate of death in the same hospital over the past several years. We would also need to know the profiles of the patients who came through the hospital's doors. How severe was their disease? What was their risk of death? What was their socio-economic background? What was their gender? All these factors loom very large in determining outcomes, even before patients receive any care at all. Attempts to build these risk-adjusted factors into determining outcomes have so far met with only partial success.[45] It is very difficult to do.

Finally, death rates seem remarkably insensitive to quite wide variations in the quality of care.[46] Often, what health-care professionals do is not closely related to the outcome they get. Teachers face the same problem. In addition, and here the web of accountability becomes even more tangled, patient motivation and behaviour is partly responsible for health-care outcomes, just as student motivation is partly responsible for educational outcomes. Analysis of outcomes, or results, can take us only so far.

Measuring effective performance is easier when we shift from results to the process of care. These kinds of measures are also more useful if the purpose of measurement is to influence what health-care professionals do. Processes are, after all, under the control of the health-care provider, while outcomes often are not. Care can be overused, underused, and misused. It is overused when health care is provided when inappropriate; it is underused when it is not provided when necessary; and it is misused when the wrong kind of health care is provided. Overuse, not surprisingly, has been the biggest concern of governments because of the consequences for costs, even though underuse and misuse can compromise quality care just as seriously as overuse.

The first and most immediate question is, Did the health-care professional do the right thing? Did we get the right treatment when we were in hospital? Were the best practices followed? More and more patients are asking, Why do the rates for certain procedures vary so widely? Why does one hospital do three times as many hysterectomies as another? How do I know how good my doctor is? Patients would be astonished to know that as many as 80 percent of medical decisions are still based on trial and error, rather than on best practices informed by research.[47] This, by the way, is not so different from education, where teachers draw on experience gained through trial and error to tailor their methods to particular groups of students.

To improve practice, governments and professionals have come together to establish clinical guidelines based on the best available knowledge. Practitioners and experts admit that knowledge is incomplete, but they survey the best available evidence and attempt to establish best practices, given what is known. This kind of evidence-based practice is more systematic than individual trial-and-error experimentation by practitioners. We can establish benchmarks for clinical practice that practitioners can use to guide what they do.

Even this kind of process is controversial. As one health-care practitioner recently explained, and exclaimed, "I simply don't believe the evidence. I trust my own judgment and experience."[48] Seasoned teachers often make the same claim when they respond to the latest study of the effectiveness of educational methods. Success with evidence-based practice in education and health care is still modest.[49] "The world wants the health-care system to have evidence-based practice," explained Carole Estabrooks of the Canadian Centre for Health Research and Policy. "And everyone says, 'Do it,' but they don't know how."[50] The identification of best practices, and compliance and monitoring by the health-care community, has been painfully slow. In some senses, health care, like education, is just moving into the post-industrial age.

2) **Efficiency.** Considerations of cost loom much larger in health care than they do in public education. It is no surprise, therefore, that hospitals, unlike schools, have been held accountable for their efficiency, and that incentives have been put in place to reward the efficient.[51] In many provinces in Canada, as well as in Great Britain and New Zealand, patients entering the hospital are weighted by their age and gender and the type and severity of their illness.[52] Average lengths of stay have been established, using the kind of evidence that is at the core of the controversies in evidence-based medicine. It seems that it is easier to use knowledge when the purpose is efficiency

rather than when it is effectiveness of care. That efficiency can never be measured appropriately unless we know what is effective often seems to be beside the point.

Hospitals that meet their targets and move people through more quickly than expected are given additional funds at the end of the fiscal year. My mother re-enters the story here. When she exceeded the expected length of stay for a geriatric patient with a broken hip, she became a problem. She became a problem even though she had a remarkable surgeon and she subsequently walked. However, she was beyond the acceptable statistical norm; she simply took "too long" to recover.

This measure of efficiency allows hospitals to treat more patients at roughly the same cost, but efficiency comes at a price. The improvement in the efficiency of hospitals has come from the capacity to discharge patients much more quickly. As a result, costs have shifted to other parts of the health-care system, and even out of the health-care system completely — to families and individuals, to your home and mine.[53] When community care, prescription drugs, and home care are publicly insured, some of the costs are publicly absorbed. When they are not publicly insured — and often they are not — families and individuals, private insurers, and voluntary organizations have paid the costs of nursing help and pharmaceuticals. The growing share of private spending in Canada's health-care system reflects this shifting of costs from the acute-care sector. Greater efficiency in the acute-care sector has led to what has accurately been called the passive privatization of the health-care system.

3) **Satisfaction.** Hospitals, like public schools, have recently begun to measure the satisfaction of their consumers. This is a measure of accountability that fits with our growing consumer culture and the emergence of markets for public goods. Canada has lagged behind health-care systems in Great Britain and the United States in "grading" its hospitals on patient satisfaction. It was only a few years ago that the Ontario Hospital Association first commissioned report cards on the province's hospitals. Patients are interviewed, the hospitals are ranked, the scores are averaged in five categories, and the results are published in local newspapers.[54] Here, too, as in schools, hospitals are compared with one another, and some are always below average. We don't know whether patients are generally satisfied with the care they've received in hospitals, only which hospitals are the best and the worst and which are "average" at satisfying their patients. Some hospitals, like some schools, will always do badly.

Not surprisingly, some people are as sceptical about the importance of patient satisfaction as a measure of hospital performance as they are about parent satisfaction as a measure of school performance. "It is possible for patients to be highly satisfied with care that kills you and to be very dissatisfied with care that saves your life," one health-care expert acidly observed.[55] Evidence has grown, however, that patient satisfaction is an important contributor to a sense of efficacy, and to patients following the instructions they are given. More important, it is a matter, as I have argued, of basic human dignity.

An important dimension in patient satisfaction with the care they receive in hospital is their access to care — the length of time they wait to get in and the length of time they wait once they are in. Waiting lists and waiting times are the public's quick barometer of the health of the health-care system. It is the citizen-consumer's hot button.

The extent and scope of waiting lists and the appropriateness of waiting times in the medical-care sector is a subject of fierce analytical and political debate.[56] There is no agreed-upon method to construct these lists, and information-management systems are not adequate to track the extent of the problem. The very limited evidence suggests both that waiting lists are getting shorter in some places for some kinds of cases and that they are getting longer in other places for other kinds of cases.[57] A systematic study of waiting lists for surgery for patients with cancer in Ontario concluded that 37 percent of patients experienced inappropriate delays.[58] Even though there is not yet reliable evidence that these kinds of delays result in worse clinical outcomes, patients at the very least experienced serious psychosocial stress. It is difficult to establish both the clinical impact of delay and accurate estimates of the size of waiting lists, partly because of how politicized reports of waiting lists are. Health-care providers have every incentive to exaggerate their length, and governments and purchasers of care have every incentive to minimize the problem.

Waiting times are somewhat easier. A nice example of a performance measure is the way hospitals in the United

Kingdom are given one to five stars for how well they meet their time targets in treating patients. The Patients Charter in Great Britain specifies standards of waiting times in clinics and hospitals. A measure of performance — which may sound almost surreal to Canadians — requires hospital staff to see a patient within five minutes of coming to an emergency room; seriously injured or sick people must be seen immediately. Report cards on the hospitals measure time between entry and contact with a health-care professional, and hospitals that receive fewer than three stars usually have to explain to their boards their failure to meet the standard — and must remedy the problem.[59] With this kind of standard, no hospital need fail, and there is follow-through when hospitals do not meet expected standards of performance.

4) **Public accountability through transparency.** No matter what measures are used, the chain of accountability is broken if results are not reported to us in ways that we as citizens can understand. In the past decade, some progress has been made in holding hospitals and physicians publicly accountable for their practices, but we in Canada are far from where we want to be.

In Scotland, for example, if you have one of four different kinds of cancer and are looking for treatment, you can find out exactly which hospitals have the best five-year survival rates.[60] New York and Pennsylvania legally mandate hospitals to provide information on how well physicians are performing surgeries, what their complication rates are, and how often patients are readmitted to

hospital after treatment. Patients are able to get very specific information about the records of both the hospital
and the doctor in treating the medical problem they have.[61]

Canada's physicians and hospitals generally have not
kept pace. Suppose for a moment that the management of
waiting lists has improved. You are waiting for cardiac
surgery and are given the option of a surgeon whose
waiting list is shorter. You don't know this doctor and
want some information about her skills and performance.
Getting that information is a struggle. In Canada, there
are no mandatory procedures in place for the disclosure
of medical error, and it is extremely difficult for patients
to get information about a physician's record of error.
Patients in Canada face many of the same problems when
they try to get information about a hospital's record on
specific procedures. Again, the problem is not the lack of
information, but its availability to the public.[62] Only
recently have Canadians begun to get easily understandable report cards on the performance of their hospitals.

Self-regulation by the professions is simply not working well enough, because it is not transparent enough.[63] A
recent report on standards of public accountability for
physicians concluded that current restrictions on inform-
ing the public are inappropriate. "It is not sufficient for
public bodies to simply do the right thing," the report
argues. "Public accountability now requires that public
bodies communicate publicly how they are in fact fulfilling their obligations."[64] The report recommended that
members of the public make up the majority of board
members of the College of Physicians and Surgeons,

which governs physician behaviour in Ontario, a recommendation that the college fiercely opposed.[65] This opposition strikes a discordant note in our ears; the medieval guild is a very poor fit, not only with the post-industrial citizen, but also with the smart state.

It need not be this way. In the state of Massachusetts, the complete histories of the 30,000 practising physicians are posted on a web site. The site includes disciplinary action by the licensing boards, hospital sanctions, malpractice settlements, and civil and criminal rulings. Patients use the web site; it has had about 7 million hits in the past four years. If you want details about every patient complaint and full discipline orders, you simply make a toll-free telephone call. "We were warned," said Nancy Sullivan, the director of the Medical Board, "that expanding public access to physician information would be too difficult, too costly, and potentially harmful to physicians."[66] It was none of these. The web site took only eight months' work by three staff, at a cost of only $300,000, and was praised by the National Academy of Sciences as a model for patient-safety programs.

When we compare accountability in education and health care, the double standards are astonishing. Teachers in the public education system across North America are now subject to testing for competency — a hotly controversial issue and an object of deep resentment — but doctors who perform the most dangerous kind of surgery are not.[67] The difference in the mechanism of accountability for teachers and doctors is striking: the government leads accountability in public education, while physicians police themselves. It is a difference that is hard to understand — and impossible to justify — given what is at stake for the public.

The Smart State and Accountability

States are more, not less, important in the post-industrial age. The post-industrial state is changing the way public goods are delivered, but it cannot — and should not — shed its fundamental accountability to all its citizens. The new smarter state can address the new agenda of accountability in very different ways. It can impose standards or take the lead in shaping new conversations to construct accountability.

Governments can simply cut costs, contract out service delivery, and eliminate existing programs to go around organized stakeholders. They can then impose standards by mandating hospital scorecards, clinical guidelines, and standards for educational testing. We have seen a great deal of that recently, although far more in public education than in health care. Alternatively, governments can change the structure of the system, as proponents of choice advocate, and leave accountability to the market. We have also seen some of that. A third possibility is that the state can negotiate the construction of accountability with unions; with non-governmental organizations, which are increasingly monitoring the performance of education and health-care delivery; with private-sector firms that are coming into public markets; and with professional associations.[68]

The difference will be significant. The voices of those

who are to be held accountable are essential. The voices of citizens in the community, who are holding providers of public goods accountable, are also essential. An open, democratic process to construct the content of accountability — what accountability means, how it is measured, and to whom providers are accountable — is no less than what citizens deserve and expect. It is also the best — indeed the only — hope governments have for active, engaged providers that are committed to the delivery of high-quality public goods. Accountability works best when local opinion leaders — the principal and teachers in the local public school, the physicians and nurses in the hospital, the physiotherapist in the community clinic — champion and explain the goals and the purposes.[69] A negotiated process of accountability is time-consuming, expensive, and difficult, but only this kind of process stands a chance of providing the quality of public goods that governments and citizens repeatedly say they want, and that providers say they want to deliver.

But voice alone will not be enough. Accountability does not take place in a social and political vacuum. It must also be negotiated within the broader context of cost-effectiveness, which governs the delivery of public goods when resources are not infinite. If citizens are rightly holding their providers and their governments accountable for the quality of the public goods that they deliver, they cannot expect shortened waiting lists, short waiting times, effective care, and outstanding educational achievement within a budgetary envelope that remains constant. If providers are expected to innovate, they must have the resources to do so. Accountability without responsiveness is meaningless, but responsiveness requires a willingness by governments — and even more so by citizens — to invest in the improvement of the public goods that they value most. Accountability is reciprocal and mutually obligating.

Voice is not enough for a second reason. It is not enough because individual and collective constructions of accountability do not always, or even often, fit comfortably together. One director of quality assurance, who is charged with assuring all these meanings of quality simultaneously in his hospital, attempted to cut through the thicket of the at times competing obligations, coming down squarely in favour of a restricted vision of state-led accountability to the broad public. "One issue of concern," he argued, "is that hospital administrators often confuse discussions of accountability by equating the needs of individual patients, who may wish simply to make 'informed choices,' with the responsibilities and due diligence that must be exercised by our legislators, who are entrusted to act on behalf of all citizens and who, at least in theory, ought to represent some broader public interest. I . . . suggest that our only true accountability lies to our legislators."[70]

Governments are indeed responsible for the quality of public goods available to all citizens. They are responsible for equitable access to public goods in societies that value fairness. In post-industrial societies, the voice for equitable access increasingly struggles to be heard among the voices for choice. This conversation is part of the long-standing tension between individual rights and collective public goods. This conversation goes beyond efficiency, and even beyond accountability, and is the one we join in the final chapter.

V

THE CULTURE OF CHOICE

The real trouble with this world of ours is not that it is an unreasonable one, nor even that it is a reasonable one. The commonest kind of trouble is that it is nearly reasonable, but not quite. Life is not an illogicality; yet it is a trap for logicians. It looks a little more mathematical and regular than it is; its exactitude is obvious, but its inexactitude is hidden; its wildness lies in wait.

— G. K. Chesterton[1]

OUR DISSECTION OF THE cult of efficiency in the post-industrial age has uncovered three unexpected paradoxes. These paradoxes tell us a great deal about our evolving society, about the new face we want our governments to show to us as citizens, and about how we imagine ourselves.

The first paradox is one that we have already explored. It is the seeding of a powerful language of accountability within our conversation about efficiency.

We turn away from the state to markets for efficiency, but we turn back again even more sharply to the state to insist on accountability. We demand that the state assure us of the quality of the public goods that these markets provide. It seems that the escape from the state in the post-industrial age is illusory. The face of the state is changing, but we want to see more of the new face, not less.

The second paradox lies deeper beneath the surface. Efficiency and markets have enabled a growing conversation about choice. We make the strongest possible claims to choice because we speak of choice as a right. We no longer speak of the freedom to choose, but of the right to choice. Here, too, as we turn away from the state to create public markets, we turn back forcefully to claim choice as an entitlement that is provided by the state. We want not only a minimalist state that guarantees the quality of our public goods, but also a state that provides entitlement to choose among public goods, and that sets appropriate rules for choice. Despite our distrust of government, our escape from the sclerotic state is more apparent than real. We want to see the state as much more than a guarantor of the quality of public goods: we want the state to provide the right to choose from among the public goods it guarantees. As citizens who prize autonomy, we are nevertheless giving the state a strong face.

The third paradox is found within our language and thinking about choice. In post-industrial society, we speak a great deal about choice and satisfaction. Even though we value choice, the way we think about it hides many of our most intractable value conflicts. We examine what is exact, as G. K. Chesterton observed, but we mask what is inexact. In so doing, we deny many of our deepest conflicts about the fundamental values that underlie difficult decisions about public goods. The content of our public conversation with one another, as citizens, and between citizens and the state, is diminished.

The Turn to Accountability

In the post-industrial age, efficiency has become an end, a value in its own right. "We are an efficient society," proudly asserts the author of a recent book about Canada. "We have seen the future, and it is . . . efficient."[2] That claim says it all. We no longer, as we did even three decades ago, proclaim the justice of our society, or its equity, or its excellence. The dogma is simple: efficiency grows out of the competition that markets bring, and accountability comes through the survival of the fittest in the market. For the high priests of efficiency, the conversation ends here. There is nothing more to talk about. What we are efficient at is discussed less and less often, and sometimes not at all. When efficiency becomes an end instead of a means, a value along with all other values, our public conversation is impoverished. Efficiency has become a cult.

If we could simply dismiss efficiency from our public conversation, the cult would have limited resonance. It would appeal only to those who distrust the state, who are deeply sceptical of its capacity to manage well, and who believe that the Weberian state is not rational, but sclerotic. "Whatever government runs, it runs badly" is the core belief that drives the cult of efficiency in public life. But we cannot dismiss efficiency from our public conversation.

We ignore efficiency at our peril. Efficiency, properly understood, is a means, not an end; a process, not a value. It is a vital tool to achieve other public goals and goods. If we are to provide the highest-quality public goods that reflect our civic values, we have no choice but to become efficient in the process. Public conversation about efficiency must move from cult to analysis, from end to means, from value to process.

Beyond the cult is a legitimate and important discussion of efficiency as cost-effectiveness in the delivery of public goods. What distinguishes the legitimate conversation from the cult is a serious and deep discussion of purpose: at what do we want to be effective? Whether this purpose is itself a route to a larger end — whether a civic education is a step toward a civic democracy or universal health care is part of a society that values fairness — does not materially affect the argument. Without discussion of purpose, effectiveness makes no sense, and without discussion of effectiveness, efficiency is stripped of its analytic power and becomes a cult.

It is no surprise that leaders across the political divide have turned to the market to look for answers. Private markets, when they are properly regulated by states, have indeed improved efficiency and created wealth. Some of this wealth has, over time, been redistributed by the state to create public goods. From private markets, political leaders drew the idea of creating markets for public goods. The new post-industrial state is the handmaiden of public markets that stimulate competition and efficiency for public goods. The idea is simple — and seductive.

Ideas, no matter how simple, elegant, and logical, often translate into messy, complicated, and even perverse practices. What happens when ideas are put into practice matters, and matters a great deal. Public markets for public goods, we have found, do not deliver what they promise. This is no surprise. Utopias, when they are made real, are always flawed. The jury is still out, and the experiment is still ongoing, but what we know is that creating a public market and changing the incentives have not yet provided clear and unmistakable gains in efficiency in the provision of public goods.

To explain the disappointing results, supporters of market models claim, as they always have, that politics continually get in the way — but politics are an inescapable part of the landscape of public goods. They cannot be wished away. Critics of market models claim, as they always do, that markets cannot provide public goods in a way that is consistent with social values. Markets are never expected to provide equity — or any other social value — only surpluses that can then be redistributed in a way that is consistent with civic values.

Putting public education and health care under the microscope tells us more than the often-polemical debate between defenders of markets and states reveals. Competition, the basic driver of efficiency, can take us only so far when the goods are public, not private. It can never be the whole answer. When the goods we are talking about are public, the language of competition is balanced and softened by the imperatives of cooperation. Markets need states to establish the framework that regulates exchanges, to protect against catastrophic market failure, and to soften the impact of competition among purchasers and providers of public goods. States need public markets to allow them to steer rather than to row, to set and monitor policy rather than to micromanage. Just as the rational state, with its bureaucratic micromanagement, is no longer satisfactory to citizens in post-industrial society, so the logic of the "survival of the fittest" when goods are public does not sit well with the values that define contemporary society.

The emergence of public markets for public goods opens a new conversation that goes beyond efficiency. Its most important contribution may be the creation of a new agenda of accountability in the post-industrial state. Competition is far from the whole answer, and accountability supplies an important missing piece. Accountability moves the focus of the debate between markets and states, between consumers and citizens. The language of accountability uses a vocabulary that transcends the ideological divide between markets and states. It softens market logic and hardens our expectations of what states must provide.

Accountability focuses on incentives as well as on standards of behaviour, on how providers of public goods can be motivated to do what is necessary and right as well as on an examination of whether they actually meet standards. This conversation also implicates purposes and fundamental values. Bundled into the story of standards and incentives are the measures we develop to evaluate performance once the standards are in place. What we count matters. The choice of measures very much depends not only on what we are measuring, but why we are measuring. Counting requires political decisions about what matters, what is included and excluded, what should be in and what should be out. The political judgements behind these decisions are implicit rather than explicit, but they shape the story the measures then tell.

Would that it were so easy. In private markets, accountability is not a logical problem. It emerges naturally through competition and the incentives that competition creates. Markets as a whole need only hard budgets. They need to know what is profitable, not what is effective. Firms within the market are different. In the equation of cost and effectiveness, they are much more interested in effectiveness. If they are to compete and survive over the long term, the quality of what they provide must improve all the time. Consumers are demanding even more. Not only do they want quality from producers, but they are also holding private firms responsible for the consequences of the products they sell: car and cigarette manufacturers are just two examples. We are adding yet one more layer of accountability; as citizens, we are increasingly holding corporations accountable for socially responsible behaviour.[3]

If we are holding corporations accountable in new ways, as citizens we have a greater right to hold our governments accountable. In post-industrial politics, citizens are more than ever tuning out conventional forms of political participation. The last elections in Britain and Canada, for example, saw the lowest turnouts of voters in modern history — this despite deep concern among voters in both countries about the quality of basic public goods and services. Some despair completely of the democratic project as it is currently formulated. In increasingly complex post-industrial societies, with their deepening social fragmentation, argues Danilo Zolo, a critic of contemporary society, "it is the democratic encyclopedia as a whole that seems designed for obsolescence, along with its most basic paradigms: participation, representation, competitive pluralism."[4]

Beneath the apathy are fundamental changes in the role of the state within society, and in the balance between individual and society. The smart state is no longer manager, but is rather regulator and standard-setter. A new equilibrium of social power is growing between the individual and society, and as journalist Philip Allott argues, public decision making is becoming a permanent dialogue rather than the periodic delegation that Weber wanted, and that we came to know throughout much of the past century.[5] In this permanent dialogue, we expect direct public accountability from those who provide our most basic public goods. We want to know who is performing effectively. And we hold our governments responsible.

The turn to accountability takes us a large step beyond the cult of efficiency. It nests efficiency within a larger discourse that uses the language of democracy as much as the language of the market. Whatever markets are, they are not democratic. Accountability is a promising terrain for public conversation because it transcends the debate between states and markets, a debate that is increasingly hollow. But — and there is always a "but" when we move beyond utopias and cults — the meaning and terms of accountability are fundamentally contested.

The "what" of accountability reflects political values. Although the polemics revolve around measures, that is not what the debates are about. Hidden beneath the polemics are arguments about goals and values. Measures, as we saw in chapter 4, always serve as surrogates for political conflict about much deeper values. The fundamental issues in any conflict over policy come alive in how we choose to count the dimensions of the problem.

What we put into the basket of accountability, and how we choose the measures, becomes the test of the permanent dialogue in the post-democratic state in the post-industrial age. Our world, G. K. Chesteron wrote a century ago, "looks a little more mathematical and regular than it is; its exactitude is obvious, but its inexactitude is hidden; its wildness lies in wait."[6] As we construct a more demanding architecture of accountability, we need to understand clearly why we are counting what we are counting, who chooses the measures and how they are chosen, how the measurers and the measures are politically connected, and what incentives these measures will create.

With a deeper and richer discussion, political conversation about accountability will take us much further than efficiency, but still not as far as we need to go. Political leaders often prefer to put the debates that engage our most important and contested values into a supposedly neutral measuring cup. They do so to mask the underlying differences in values and purposes, and to dampen political disagreements. They seek the consensus they need and the political protection they want by transforming conflict over purpose into discussion of measures, and in the process they hide and evade differences about values and goals. But there is no simple scientific or quantitative fix to the political process of constructing accountability: numbers cannot bear the political burden they are being asked to carry. There is no escape from an admittedly difficult conversation about our values and purposes. The core question remains, Accountability for what?

The Culture of Choice in Post-industrial Society

When we listen closely to our contemporary discussion about public goods, we hear yet one more debate that is emerging explicitly in public conversation, and it is about choice. Conversation about choice and its limits takes us directly to a discussion of our civic values. Before we consider how a growing culture of choice bumps up against other cultures and values, how it is rotating the axis of our public conversation, we need to turn our attention to its roots.

Why do we talk about choice more now than ever before? What is it about post-industrial society that fuels a culture of choice? Choice, after all, has been fundamental to democratic life for centuries, but largely as an instrument to achieve other ends that we value. Why do we so often hear language that places inherent value on the right to choice?

Choice is a luxury of an affluent society, comfortable and secure in its economic future. Notwithstanding the graphic threat of terrorism in North America, our post-industrial society is the first in historical memory to enjoy existential security; collective survival is not an immediate issue burnt into public consciousness. Most people alive today do not enjoy this privileged condition. They struggle in poverty for survival from war and disease in a climate of overwhelming insecurity. They do not talk much about choice. In post-industrial, affluent, and secure society, the right to choose figures prominently in the foreground because the background is still and quiescent, at least for the majority of citizens. Talk about choice grows out of the comfortable silence.

It is no surprise that those who are better off generally tend to value choice and those who are disadvantaged tend to value equity through redistribution from the stronger to the weaker, the richer to the poorer. This is true for individuals and for societies — citizens in Greece, as I mentioned earlier, are more willing to support redistribution than are citizens of Canada, where the standard of living and the quality of life are significantly higher. That affluence excludes a significant minority within post-industrial society does not dampen talk about choice by the affluent majority. The social consensus around redistribution created during the late industrial era, when budgets were growing and demands were more limited, fractured during a period of deficit reduction and retrenchment. This consensus has splintered completely in the post-industrial era. It is unlikely that the old social consensus can be stitched together again — and certainly not in the same way.

It is not only affluence that fosters a culture of choice, but also the new forms of economic and social organization in post-industrial society. Much has been written about our consumer society, its glorification of material pleasures, and its endless stimulation of public wants — wants, not needs — through advertising. This is hardly new. It was characteristic of industrial capitalism. What *has* changed is the capacity of post-industrial society to stoke individual wants and then customize their satisfaction. Henry Ford's assembly line lowered the cost and increased the effectiveness of the automobile, but it did so by narrowing choice. "Any customer," he offered, "can have a car painted any color that he wants as long as it is black."[7] Now we can design a car, or a computer, or a course, or a house, through the World Wide Web. Digital technology and private markets are multiplying the choices consumers have and giving them the autonomy to customize what they want. Private markets now give pride of place to diversity, customization, autonomy, and choice. As Adam Smith's pin factory becomes more difficult to find in our economic landscape, the widening gap between the customization of private goods and the homogenization of public goods is fuelling the culture of choice in public life in affluent societies.

Reinforcing the culture of choice is the widespread decline of deference to established authority. It is not only political leaders who are the object of growing distrust and cynicism, but also religious leaders, union leaders, medical authorities, and educators. Watergate, not Vietnam, asserts a colleague, was the defining moment in the creation of post-industrial politics in North America. Distrust of authority leads to a growing unwillingness to delegate decision-making powers on issues that we consider important. It also leads to an assertion of the right to choice, to reclaim authority that might well be misused. It is not, as Joseph Heath has argued, efficiency that has displaced religion, ethnicity, and language as the source of public loyalty.[8] It is, rather, autonomy and self-assertion that have replaced loyalty and deference to public authorities. The assertion of the right to choice is the voice citizens raise against authority that they increasingly distrust.

Finally, the new importance of knowledge in the post-industrial economy gives weight to the language of choice. The raw material of production in post-industrial society, as we have seen, is knowledge. Knowledge, thought, and creativity empower not only in work, Antonio Negri concludes, but in life.[9] If knowledge, thinking, innovation, and creativity are the privileged attributes in private life, they cannot long be segregated from public life. Knowledge joins with a decline of deference to authority, takes root in affluence, and blows on the winds of customization and diversity to provide fertile breeding grounds for a culture of choice.

The culture of choice fits comfortably with the radical individualism that is increasingly the hallmark of affluent post-industrial societies. We have seen that although public markets in education and health care do not deliver the efficiencies they have promised, they remain seductive as instruments to deliver public goods. Their attraction is puzzling until their lustre is embedded in the culture of choice that reflects post-industrial politics and society. The widespread emphasis on expressivism, autonomy, and self-realization across post-industrial politics and society finds resonance in the language of choice. The weight of the individual and society is once again in the process of being rebalanced.

Choice is fundamental to the political language of those who look to markets as models for the configuration of public space. It is also part of the vocabulary of those who celebrate the end of industrial capitalism, the emergence of the knowledge-based economy, and the shift from representative democracy, which forces one-size-fits-all solutions on diverse populations, to a new politics of expression. Choice is becoming part of the discourse of a new left-wing politics that revolves around liberty and the quality of life rather than around the "reductive quest for equality between groups."[10] We should not be surprised that choice is bubbling up as part of our post-industrial conversation. The nineteenth century, argues social commentator Alan Wolfe, was about economic freedom. The twentieth century was about political freedom. This century will be about individual freedom; individuals will determine for themselves what it means to live a good and virtuous life.[11]

The Freedom to Choose and the Limits to Choice

As the culture of choice broadens and deepens, we speak more and more about the right to choice and less and less about the freedom to choose. That language is especially curious because liberty, as the focus of public conversation, is where the tensions between individual autonomy and purpose and collective consequences have historically played most vividly.

This changing discourse is no accident. There are important degrees of difference between the freedom to choose and the right to choice. The right to choice makes a much stronger claim than does the freedom to choose. While both implicate the state, the language of freedom treats the state as intrusive and seeks to restrict its role. The vocabulary of rights, on the other hand, makes a claim on the state and imposes an obligation. The state here is not shy and retiring. It cannot stay in the background, but instead must step forward to meet its obligations.

Our contemporary discussion of the right to choice connects in part to earlier conversations about liberty. Choice and liberty are often conflated, but they are not one and the same. "The rock climber on a difficult pitch who sees only one way out to save his life is unquestionably free," argues Hayek, "though we would hardly say he has any choice."[12] Liberty is, however, a precondition of meaningful choice. If we are coerced or manipulated, we do not have the capacity to make meaningful choice. We do not want to be coerced into making a choice, even when the choice we are pressured to make is the choice that we would have made anyway.[13] Restrictions on liberty, therefore, speak indirectly to restrictions on choice.

Individual liberty has never been, nor could it be, wholly unrestricted. In his classic essay *On Liberty*, John Stuart Mill put very few limits on individual liberty: "The only purpose for which power can be rightfully exercised over any member of a civilized community, against his will, is to prevent harm to others."[14] Mill, and many others who followed, gave maximum scope to individual liberty, short of causing harm to others. But what constitutes harm? It is how we answer this question that shapes how we think about collective restrictions on liberty, and about restrictions on individual choice, for Mill connected liberty closely to the availability of choice.[15]

The answer to this question is still being vigorously argued. Physical harm, material harm, environmental harm, psychological harm, social harm, and community harm are all grist for the mill in the debate about the appropriate limits to individual choice. We heard echoes of this debate in chapter 3 when we examined the consequences of school choice for civic democracy and its shared ideals. Those supporting choice do not consider the damage that may be done to shared civic ideals — and to the children who remain in the public schools — sufficiently harmful to restrict choice. Those opposed to choice think that the harm that will be inflicted through the loss of the shared experience in community schools is sufficient to restrict the freedom to choose. The principle of "do no harm" takes us only so far, for it is the meaning we give to "harm" that continues to shape our contemporary debates about markets and states.[16]

The meaning we give to harm is not static, but changes as our societies, our cultures, and our politics evolve. Our definition of harm has grown as we have come to know more about the social, cultural, environmental, and political conditions that can do harm. Socio-economic status, as we know, is the strongest predictor of health and individual achievement. As our knowledge of harm expands, we are led to place greater restrictions on individual choice that contributes to these harms. The boundaries of liberty have narrowed in knowledge-based, post-industrial society. Yet citizens in post-industrial societies give greater weight to individual autonomy within society than we did even fifty years ago. We do so because most of us are generally more affluent, more comfortable, more knowledgeable, and certainly much more distrustful of authority.

Post-industrial society creates paradoxes for the scope we give to liberty. We have learned that to make choices, we must be enabled by the conditions under which we live. Here, too, strong arguments can be made for the creation of the social conditions that enhance people's capacity to make choices. This holds especially for choice among public goods; public goods like education and health care have become fundamental to an individual's capacity to make autonomous choice. In post-industrial society, the contradictions have sharpened: we value the liberty to make choices more, but we know far better than we ever have that the social context of choice matters. The dilemmas of liberty and its restrictions are consequently more acute.

The Right to Choose: Possibility and Commitment

The language of liberty is not the only language that citizens in post-industrial society speak. We also speak increasingly about the right to choice. A rights claim is the strongest kind of claim that we can make, because it entails entitlement and obligation by others. When we as citizens claim the right to choose among public goods, we are no longer claiming freedom from the state. On the contrary, we are insisting that the state actively provide meaningful choice among public goods. Here, too, the contradictions in post-industrial society have sharpened. As citizens who are increasingly distrustful of the state, we value autonomy, yet we claim the right to choice, a claim that obligates the state in new ways. We want it both ways: we want a state that will turn its face away, and we want a state with the capacity to provide choice in public goods.

The rights revolution, as Michael Ignatieff reminds us, has been gathering steam for the past half century. Although the revolution has momentum, rights everywhere remain politically contested. Rights do not derive from the state: some argue that they derive simply from being human, others embed them in natural rights, still others in principles of right and wrong, and some derive rights from rationality. How different societies understand rights, what content they give to them, what rights are claimed, what rights are enforced by the state, what obligations rights create, and what consequences flow from rights are the subjects of heated political debate. This is, of course, not a new debate. The likelihood that rights will submit to a simple set of shared meanings in the post-industrial age is low. This, too, is a deeper debate about values, embedded in different cultural traditions and institutional histories.

To talk about rights, we need first to distinguish between procedural and substantive rights.[17] Procedural rights spell out an explicit process through which decisions must be made. Guarantees of trial by a jury of peers, freedom from arbitrary arrest and imprisonment, freedom from torture — these are procedural rights. These rights are familiar to the fortunate who live in liberal democratic societies, and they are fundamental to their capacity to shape the institutions of governance and to hold accountable those they choose to invest with legitimate authority. The right to choose leaders through fair processes, for example, and to hold them accountable, is a fundamental procedural right. Once these rights are recognized, they imply a rule of both law and equity, for a right for one is a right for all.

Substantive rights go beyond procedures to specify entitlements. Freedoms of speech, of assembly, and of religion are widely accepted substantive rights in liberal democratic societies. We speak of these as negative substantive rights — the right to do something free of restraint.[18] Positive substantive rights are even more demanding. They are rights to have or receive something, and these rights are coupled with the duties of others. These kinds of rights are even more deeply contested because they create obligations for others. It is here that the right to choice bumps up, uneasily, against other rights.

In the past three decades, a growing chorus of voices has argued that if people lack the material means to exercise their procedural and substantive rights, these rights scarcely matter. Take, for example, access to public education. If citizens have no education, if they are not literate, it becomes far more difficult to exercise the right to free speech and political assembly. India, the great experiment in mass democracy, has worked its way around these obstacles, but few would dispute the proposition that an educated citizenry can more effectively exercise its procedural and substantive rights. Public education has been widely recognized as a positive substantive right because it implicates other rights.

Much the same holds for health. The central importance of health to the exercise of autonomous choice has made it a positive substantive right.[19] The right to health has been recognized globally by the World Health Organization in its groundbreaking report *Health for All*, and in the growing emphasis on patients' charters, which explicitly use the language of rights to specify patient entitlements. Great Britain has a very specific patients' charter that establishes general rights and particular entitlements. Although honoured far more in the breach than in the observance — no different from other substantive and procedural rights in many parts of the world — the substantive right to health reflects the realization that the ill who are denied care cannot exercise any of their procedural or substantive rights in a democratic society.

Rights to education and health are fundamentally social and political. Rights cannot be exercised in a vacuum; they require social and political supports. Society is constitutive of the exercise of any individual right — procedural or substantive. "The social cannot be reduced to the individual," argues the philosopher Roy Bhaskar. "It is equally clear that society is a necessary condition for any intentional human acts at all."[20] Social values directly affect the capacity of individuals to exercise their rights, just as the exercise of rights implicates society. This is particularly so for substantive rights. We cannot understand the current dilemmas surrounding public goods without an appreciation of the social supports that make it possible for some people to exercise those rights and the social obstacles that make it difficult, if not impossible, for others. The exercise of these rights has fundamental implications for the way that social values are interpreted. There is a gap — at times small and at times large — between the discourse of rights and rights practice.

If the rights revolution has been about both enhancing our right to be equal and protecting our right to be different, as Michael Ignatieff argues, then the right to be different implies the right to choose.[21] Choice has long been part of public as well as private conversation, not as a right, but largely as an instrument to achieve other ends.

Markets are inconceivable without choice. Choice is so fundamental that economists rarely make it explicit as an essential element within market logic. It is through choice, as C. B. Macpherson observed in his 1965 Massey Lectures, that the market maximizes satisfaction, but as he noted pointedly, only those satisfactions that people can afford to buy.[22]

Choice is also fundamental to liberal democratic theory and practice. The right to choose our representatives is at the core of democratic governance. It is not a sufficient condition of a mature liberal democracy, but it is absolutely necessary. A universal guarantee of the procedural rights necessary to exercise that choice, because it is foundational, is central in liberal democracies. Without these procedural guarantees, choice becomes the unmasked exercise of power. In both markets and liberal democracies, choice is the process through which other fundamental values are realized and protected. It has instrumental value.

Some of our current talk about the right to choice is different. The right to choice is used in our contemporary discussion in two distinct ways. The first, familiar to us, pays attention to the substance of choice. It looks at the substantive values at stake, requires meaningful differences among the options, and pays attention to the end results of choice. The parent who claimed the right of choice because she wanted a religious education for her child was claiming a right embedded in the language of end results and commitment.

The second is newer in our conversation. It places

inherent value — independent of the results of choice — on the right to choice. When we listened to the debate about public education in chapter 3, we heard parents assert that the right to choose their child's school is fundamental. The right was not tied to commitments or results; at issue was not whether the child performs better or worse in the chosen school, or whether one school differs significantly from another, but simply the inherent right to choice. In health care, as patients openly acknowledge, the right to choice is also fundamental. Indeed, in Canada, the patient's right to choice was one of the overarching principles of the *Medical Care Act* of 1966. Here, the language of the right to choice is about openness and possibility. The right to choice allows for the unimagined and the unanticipated, avoids closing off possibilities prematurely, and makes space for self-recreation as conditions change.[23] These two concepts of the right to choice and its limits play out very differently when we think about public goods.

Limits to the right to choice are now the subject of intense political debate, the fault line of controversy in post-industrial societies. To get a sense of the controversy, we need listen to just two quite distinct contemporary voices. One places minimal restrictions on the right to choice. The philosopher Robert Nozick establishes only two limiting conditions: the process through which choice is exercised must meet some procedural conditions, and the exercise of choice must be voluntary rather than imposed.[24] Choice as a fundamental right, as he sees it, is limited only by the conditions of choice, rather than by its results. It is truly an individual project. This is the strongest kind of claim to the right to choice that can be made, for it is unbounded by the larger social context. If the process through which I choose my child's school is appropriate and my choice is voluntary, then the substantive values embedded in the options and the consequences for the system of public education are not relevant. This kind of claim places even fewer restrictions on the right to choice than did the concept of negative liberty, which explored the harmful consequences of choice. It is unrestrained by commitment and gives pride of place to possibility. Here, the right to choice is a right against the intrusion of the state. And here, the face of the state fades.

A second voice, that of the political theorist John Rawls, puts far more stringent limits on the right to choice. Rawls writes about justice, but his concept of justice has implications for appropriate limits to the right to choice. He argues that each person should have an equal right to the most extensive basic liberty that is compatible with others. But what are the boundaries of freedom and choice? Rawls asks us all to imagine a meeting at which each of us represents future generations of our families. The purpose of our meeting is to agree on the basic principles and rules that will shape our institutions, and we must all agree that these principles are just. Using differences in power, or wealth, or race, or ethnicity, to get the principles we want would not be fair: to get around this obstacle, our conversation takes place through a veil of ignorance, where we imagine that we do not know what endowments we will have. We consequently exclude unfair advantages from our conversation and agree on the fairest possible rules.[25] We would need to agree on the principles that govern the basic structure of society, which assigns rights and duties and regulates the distribution of social and economic advantages. What kinds of principles and rules would come out of this kind of conversation?

The principle of equal liberty, the first principle, must be supplemented by principles to compensate for the social and economic inequalities and differences that restrict people's access to "social primary goods," or what we have called public goods. Why do we worry about the inequalities that restrict access to public goods? These social primary goods, Rawls answers, are enablers of choice, goods that we need in order to make meaningful choices. Education and health are essential preconditions of the capacity to exercise the right to choice; the sick and the illiterate cannot make meaningful choices. While the distribution of wealth and income need not be equal, Rawls argues, it must be to everyone's advantage. "All social values — liberty and opportunity, income and wealth, and the bases of self-respect — are to be distributed equally, unless an unequal distribution of any, or all, of these values is to everyone's advantage."[26] These principles protect against unfairness. Although Rawls does not talk explicitly about the right to choice, the implications of his argument give us pause: when we exercise our right to choice among public goods, that right is constrained by larger considerations of justice as fairness. We must consider the consequences of our choice for the distribution of social benefits that enable others to choose.[27]

These two very different approaches to the right to choice are the subject of intense political debate in our public discussions. They have profoundly different consequences for the way we think about public goods and the role of the state. The first gives us an almost unrestricted right to choice, even when goods are public, while the second limits the right to choice, especially among public goods, if the consequences of our choice would disadvantage and disable others. Each approach also has profoundly different consequences for the state. In the first, the role of the state is very limited. In the second, the state must play a far more active role in setting rules for choice that ensure justice, particularly for the disadvantaged.

These two concepts of the right to choice are not used consistently within the current ideological divide. They do not fit neatly into the camps of the political warriors in post-industrial society. Those who favour abortion, for example, describe themselves as "pro-choice," anchoring their arguments in an unrestricted right to choice. Those who oppose abortion claim the right of the unborn fetus to life, and insist that the exercise of the right to choice is constrained by its results, by the harm it does to others. They invoke the results and challenge the right to choice, even if that choice is voluntary and made in conformity with established rules. The same arguments play differently when the issue is the creation of markets for public goods. Those who favour markets assert the inherent right to choice, while those who oppose them argue that the exercise of an unrestricted right to choice will degrade public systems that are the only option available to the majority and, especially, the least advantaged. Our public talk, as we see, is inconsistent. Each of us at times invokes both arguments — an unrestricted right to choice and the results of choice — depending on the issue at stake and the values that are implicated. The issue drives the talk more than the talk drives the issue.

It is this debate about the limits to the right to choice, one that draws in part on earlier arguments about the limits to liberty, which defines the boundaries of the conversation in post-industrial society about some of our most important public goods. By invoking a right to choice, we obligate the state. We insist that the state create the conditions, set the rules, and provide public goods in such a way that we can exercise the right to choose. This rights claim is fraught with contradictions.

We are seeking from the state a right to choose a public, not a private, good. If we accept the strongest possible rights claim, we impose very few restrictions on the right to choice and limit the scope and reach of the post-industrial state. We want no more from the state than an assurance that the market is providing high-quality public goods from which we can voluntarily choose. This is the only face of the post-industrial state that some citizens want to see.

We need to remember, however, that these goods are public, that they do not exclude any citizen. Once we remember that they are public goods, then the consequences of our choice for other citizens cannot be excluded from the conversation. We cannot look only at the process of choice and satisfy ourselves that it is appropriate and that choice is voluntary. The language of possibility needs to be bounded by the language of commitment. When the goods are public, the consequences of our choice for the choices that others can make do matter. If we accept this logic, as I do, then we want more from the state than an assurance of quality. The post-industrial state is stepping back as manager; however, it is stepping forward not only as the guarantor of quality, but as the guardian of the results of the right to choice. We as citizens claim our right to choice, but we accept that it will be limited by the consequences that right imposes on others. The post-industrial state is very much present, as its predecessor was, as the trustee of fairness, equity, and justice. This is the face of the state that I as a citizen, along with many others, want to see.

Thinking about Choice: The Illusion of Solution

It is surprising, given how important choice has been to theories of both markets and liberal democracy, how little explicit attention has been paid to the way we think about choice itself. It is the largely silent partner in the conversation about markets and states. Liberalism, the foundation of much contemporary talk about democracy and markets, identifies value with what is useful to the individual. Human beings are conceived as self-interested individuals who fulfil their needs through planning and rational calculation. Choice, the result of this purposive calculation, is conspicuous by its absence. It is the utilitarians who developed systematic ways of thinking about choice.

Utilitarians look not at the conditions under which choice is made or at its results but at the inherent satisfaction that choice brings and its contribution to individual welfare. Here the focus is not on standards external to the chooser but on internal standards. This is the familiar utilitarian tradition that is silent about goals, neutral about values, and measures welfare. It starts with the preferences of those who are choosing, estimates the likely costs and benefits of the available options, and combines these estimates, using some common measure, to determine the most rational, efficient choice. Utilitarians insist that a single metric can measure and combine all the likely costs and benefits.

Without a single measuring stick, rational choice is impossible. It is this tradition that is critical to the way we think about choice today, and numbers are essential to working out the logic. Numbers offer the false promise, argues political scientist Deborah Stone, of "conflict resolution through arithmetic. . . . Once a phenomenon has been converted into a quantitative measure, it can be added, multiplied, divided, or subtracted, even though these operations have no meaning in reality. Numbers provide the comforting illusion that incommensurables can be weighed against each other, because arithmetic always 'works.' . . . Numbers force a common denominator where there is none."[28] Stone is right. The way we think about choice masks our deep conflicts about values — conflicts that are often intractable.

There is no masking, no escaping this kind of conflict. We heard echoes of conflict over values again and again as we listened to the debates about public education and health care. These kinds of conflicts cannot be resolved. They are rarely resolved even at the individual level. Modern psychology has documented the sophisticated strategies that we develop to avoid, rather than address, deep conflict among values. One of my very able students wanted to go abroad to graduate school in a specialized field, but she is the only child of a recently widowed mother. She persuaded herself that two additional years of general studies would better prepare her for more specialized work later. This is hardly a convincing argument. She rationalized a choice that engaged two competing values: her commitment to her own future and her commitment to her needy parent. We are expert at denying this kind of conflict among values.

It is much less likely that these deep value conflicts can be solved at the collective level, for at least two reasons. First, even when we make rational choices to maximize our satisfaction, we can produce collectively undesirable results. Remember our voter who, even though she valued democracy, nevertheless quite rationally chose to stay at home, to free-ride. The point, of course, is that if we all acted that way, as individuals we might benefit from not voting, from having some free time, but collectively we would suffer: our democratic processes would disappear. Second, when we use the language of rights, and make the strongest possible claims, the space for political compromise diminishes. It is easier to compromise when interests compete; we are quite adept at trading. Rights are foundational and non-negotiable. No metric, no number, can make conflicts over rights disappear, and thinking about choice in ways that promise a solution through a shared metric is a logician's trick. Life, as Chesterton told us, is indeed a trap for logicians. We can only turn back to political conversation about purpose, goals, and values, and search for a fair, if not a just, and a transient, if not a permanent, compromise.

The Value, and Illusion, of Choice

As citizens in post-industrial society, we value choice. Although it has long been part of our liberal democratic heritage, choice matters more to us now than in the past. The instrumental benefits of choice may not always be uppermost in our minds. We assert the inherent right to choice, independent of its results. A very good student of mine decided recently to apply to several graduate programs in the United States, even though he had already decided to stay in Canada and had been accepted by the leading program in his field. Puzzled, I asked him why he was bothering. The consequences were clearly not an issue, since he had already made up his mind. "I want to know," he explained, "that I have a choice." Having a choice strikes a deeper psychological chord and answers deeper needs than post-industrial economics and politics alone would suggest.

Believing that we have a choice gives us a great deal that is important to us as human beings. It speaks to our conception of ourselves as moral beings, for moral beings must have the capacity to choose. My own religious tradition locates moral behaviour in the constant struggle to choose the inclination to good in the presence of the inclination to evil. That choice is not foreordained. If we have no choice, then acting in a principled way is empty of meaning.

Believing that we have a choice also affirms our autonomy and our fundamental dignity as human beings. At the same time, it allows us greater capacity for self-expression, and for expression of our individuality, not only of what makes us human, but of what makes us different and unique as human beings. Exercising choice can be an act of self-discovery and learning. My teenage sons tell me over and again, with increasing stridency in their voices, "Let me choose. Even if I make a mistake, I want to choose for myself." They are right. The opportunity to make choices enables us to grow and develop. Even as adults, we often find that struggling with a choice can sometimes reveal what is truly important to us and what is not. We discover reasons for our decisions that had not occurred to us before we began wrestling with the choice. We learn about ourselves, our values, and our priorities.[29] At times, contrary to the dominant logic of rational choice, we make our choice first and then reason back to discover why we made the choice we did. In the process of choosing, we uncover parts of ourselves that we might have kept hidden. We find ourselves not only through abstract reasoning, but by engaging, through our emotions as well as our reason, with the choices that life presents.[30] Here choice speaks the language of possibility, exploration, creativity, and change.

Believing that we have a choice also brings an increased sense of efficacy and control. "We want to believe," argues the philosopher Claudia Mills, "that the central facts of our lives contain in them some fundamental element of our own selection and decision. . . . [W]e want to have and make choices not only because of the good results that will accrue to us in this way, but because we believe that a life in which we choose between options is better than a life in which we do not."[31]

These needs are as important in public life as they are in private life, when public goods are at stake as well as when we consider our private choices. Believing that we have a choice creates a stronger incentive to participate in public life and public conversation, and to engage with our community. The belief that we can make moral choices, a sense of autonomy and dignity, and confidence in our efficacy are all valuable and important constitutive elements of a mature civic democracy.

You may have noticed that I used the words "believing that we have a choice" as I explored the gifts that this belief brings. Again, Claudia Mills puts it eloquently: "We want a sense that we are the authors of our own lives, that our lives, if you will, are stories that we write rather than just read. We want a sense of our lives as something we do and not something that merely happens to us. . . . [But] after all, by and large, our lives *do* happen to us."[32] Possibility is bounded on one side by commitment and on the other by circumstance. We are constrained by circumstance: by chance; by our environment, our community, our society, our polity; and by large and impersonal global forces. We have little control over many of these forces, and little opportunity to write the narrative. And so, often through the illusion of choice, by believing that we have a choice, by acting as though we have a choice, we make sense of what has happened, we put our own stamp on it, and we insert our story as part of the larger shared narrative. Weaving our story into the larger narrative is an important part of constructing public life.

The difficulty arises when by telling our own story, we unfairly and rudely preempt the tales of others. Often our talk about choice is an assertion of the right to choice, with little attention paid to the results of our choice for the capacity of others to exercise their right to choice. Talk is not conversation: talk can involve only assertion, but conversation requires reasoned interaction with others in ways that do not intimidate. We hear more and more talk about the right to choice, but not enough conversation. Choice talk expressed in the language of rights does not fit comfortably with other rights already in the basket. Talk about the right to choice needs to join the conversation about other rights and the rights of others.

By exercising our right to choice, we may limit the meaningful choices of others. How do we, as a society, deal with this contradiction? The utilitarian calculus assumes that the incommensurables are somehow commensurable, that the intractable is tractable through numbers and a common yardstick. Our public discussion and our ways of thinking about choice paper over these fundamental conflicts. If, for example, the right to choice limits the rights of others to meaningful choice — if the individual's choice to exit the public system severely degrades the quality of choices for those who remain — we will have made a Faustian bargain.[33] In post-industrial society, we will have to acknowledge and live with these intractable conflicts as we continue to experiment with new ways of balancing commitment and possibility in the delivery of our most important public goods.

Americans, argues Joseph Heath, value liberty and the right to choice more than they do efficiency. The inefficiencies that follow from the unrestricted right to choice have created large social inequalities. "In many ways," Heath continues, "American civilization is like a great social experiment, designed to see just how much inefficiency people will be prepared to tolerate in the name of liberty. . . . Canadians are, in general, willing to accept such restrictions [on individual liberty], while Americans are not. This is the major reason why our society is more efficient."[34] Canadians do not value efficiency for its own sake, and the conflict of values is not a conflict between liberty and efficiency. Canadians care deeply about choice, as we have heard in the conversations about health care and education. But we have historically been willing to restrict the right to choice because we valued justice and equity more than does American society.

What matters is not only the right to choice, but the kinds of choices that we consider. Robert Reich, the former Secretary of Labor in the United States, puts it well:

I relish my freedom as much as anyone. But my freedom
isn't equivalent to the breadth or quantity of my choices.
You and I need freedom to make the significant choices —
such as what we stand for, to what and to whom we're
going to commit our lives, and what we want by way of a
community and a society. . . . [35]

The kind of balance that emerges from this conversation about the right to choice will have profound
consequences on our thinking about public goods in the
post-industrial age. A widespread right to choice within
the public system may be consistent with many — but not
all — of the values of public education, and it may bring
significant benefits to the least advantaged. Not least
among these may be an enhanced capacity to build community and the opportunity for many more to tell their
stories as part of the rich tapestry of the public narrative.
In health care, the right to choice plays differently. There
are those who argue that it is Canadians' unrestricted
right to choose a family practitioner that is creating the
"inefficiencies" in our health-care system and compro-
mising the quality of care. Improving efficiency would
constrain choice. How important to Canadians is this
individual right to choice, and how is it balanced against
the substantive right to health for all?

Choice talk is part of our larger conversation about
rights — and the values that inform these rights. The
right to choice is one right among many in the basket
of rights. How to balance rights, and the values that
inform these rights, is an age-old debate. The debate has

travelled through the centuries, from the ancient Greeks to the post-industrial age, through wave after revolutionary wave. It has led to a continuous rebalancing of the relationship between the individual and society, within changing concepts of authority and legitimacy. Expansion of the right to choice of public goods — itself inherently desirable — will have to be balanced, and balanced carefully, against the consequences for those least able to bear the costs of changes in the way public goods are delivered. Canadians, like those in many other post-industrial societies, value not only choice and all it brings with it, but also justice, fairness, and equity, however we understand and give meaning to these values.

The conflict among these values is often intractable and incommensurable. It is because these conflicts are intractable that we turn to conversation in public space, and to those we choose to govern, to set legitimate rules for a conversation that is not about interests, but about principles and values. The legitimacy of this conversation rests on recognized, fair, inclusive, and open procedures for deliberation and persuasion, where those who join in reflective discussion are neither intimidated nor manipulated.[36]

The conversation continues, with no prospect of final resolution. As citizens, we will have to acknowledge the contradictions and live with the incommensurable, even as we seek through conversation among ourselves to determine at what we want to be efficient, to give meaning to accountability and to negotiate its terms, and to rebalance rights and values in public space. We need to pay attention not only to what we can measure, but even more important, to what we cannot. Without this kind of admittedly difficult and demanding conversation about values and purposes, efficiency is reduced to a cult and accountability becomes a misleading exercise in arithmetic.

Even as we assert our right to tell our own story, we must listen attentively and fairly to the stories of others. What is important is inclusive and reflective public conversation, first about values and only then about choice, first about ends and only then about means, and first about purpose and only then about instruments. And as post-industrial society takes form and shape, as knowledge expands our sense of what is collectively possible, we will have to find new ways to bound possibility with commitment. As the one forecloses the other, possibility and commitment are always in tension with one another. The language we use to speak about this tension will test our capacity to provide both the "public" and the "good" in public goods.

POSTSCRIPT

SECURITY IN THE
POST-INDUSTRIAL AGE

As I WAS FINISHING THIS BOOK, a network of terrorists attacked the two towers of the World Trade Center in Manhattan and the Pentagon in Washington. Concerned citizens are turning to their governments to provide the most fundamental public good: security. The modern state emerged in history not through its ability to provide welfare and happiness for the greatest number of its citizens, but through its capacity to provide security. Security speaks to the most basic purpose of the state.

The state as we know it, with its monopoly on the legitimate use of force, was created through war. Three hundred years ago, as the sovereign state emerged, it grew in size and extended its reach at home by expanding its capacity to make war.[1] Throughout most of the past century, and indeed for most of recorded human history, we have lived with the fear of violent death in war. The scope of destruction that war could wreak grew over time: the unprecedented carnage of the First World War, the vicious brutality of the Second World War, and, more recently, the spectre of a nuclear holocaust foreshortened our capacity to think broadly about collective welfare. At its peak, the conflict between the superpowers threatened nuclear war and the destruction of hundreds of millions of people. Generation after generation grew up preoccupied with the possibility of catastrophic global war, and they subordinated their concerns about welfare to those of survival.

The reach and power of industrial states continued to grow as they joined in the war, first against Nazi Germany and then against the Soviet Union as the spearhead of communism. In the United States, the "imperial" presidency and the national security bureaucracy, which fought the enemy within as well as the enemy without, increased the capacity of the state to reach deeply into society and sorely tested many of the fundamental democratic values.[2] Yet as long as the prospect of global war and the extinction of the species were imaginable, the state and the protection it promised remained at the centre of politics and the object of its citizens' loyalty.

We think of the fall of the Berlin Wall in 1989 as the end of the Cold War. It signified far more, marking as sharp a divide in the twentieth century as the industrial revolution had in the nineteenth. For the first time in almost one hundred years, people living in affluent, democratic societies gained existential security; they were free of the fear that they and their societies could be obliterated through global war. Existential security is far from a global phenomenon, but it is a transformative luxury enjoyed by people living in post-industrial societies.

In the wake of the terrorist attacks in the United States, the language of war is again being spoken throughout post-industrial societies and, indeed, around the world. But a war against terrorism is a war like no other in the past century: it is not a war of states against other states, with an identifiable adversary and known targets. Far more important, terrorism does not and cannot threaten the existential security of post-industrial societies. Despite the carnage inflicted on New York and Washington, the survival of the United States or any other affluent, democratic society is not at issue. War is the wrong lens through which to view the struggle against terrorism and the language of global war is the wrong language.

The network of terror that perpetrated the attack is enabled by conditions unique to our times. Global networks of terror are conceivable only in a world that is tightly interconnected and in societies that are moving through the processes of post-industrialization. Without global markets and communications, the widespread mobility of people, and multicultural, diverse societies, these networks of terror could not survive, much less succeed.

We have witnessed the first large-scale violent attack against post-industrial society, using its characteristic form of organization: the network. The network has become the most pervasive organizational image and the dominant form of social organization in post-industrial society. "As a historical trend," observes sociologist

Manuel Castells, "dominant functions and processes in the information age are increasingly organized around networks. Networks constitute the new social morphology of our societies, and the diffusion of networking logic substantially modifies the operation and outcomes in processes of production, experience, power, and culture."[3]

Global networks are generally highly decentralized, with different leadership branches that operate with a large degree of autonomy. Unlike the tight pyramids of command-and-control structures, the hallmark of industrial society, networks are "flat," with leaders who are empowered to act under a minimum of direction and supervision. Multinational corporations, for example, or global networks of environmental groups, physicians, or journalists are generally nimble, lean, and flexible. With far-flung operations, they depend on easy mobility across porous borders.

Global networks of terror bear an uncanny resemblance to their generally benign and productive counterparts. Often with life cycles of decades, if not generations, networks of terror thrive on the openness, flexibility, and diversity of post-industrial society, crossing borders almost as easily as goods and services, knowledge, and cultures. They have global reach, particularly when they can operate within the fabric of the most open and multicultural societies, and through post-industrial organizational forms. Many also cling to host states like barnacles for the infrastructure and resources that they need; they depend on the existence of states for their own existence.[4] Unlike legitimate global networks, of course, networks of terror work in secrecy through illegitimate practices and violence to advance their political purposes. Nevertheless, it is no small irony that violent opposition to globalization and post-industrial societies takes place through a network, their signature organization.

Global networks of terror pose difficult challenges to citizens and states in affluent, democratic societies. Today citizens in post-industrial societies are turning to states to supply security from terror. But how does the new smart state provide security? How does it respond to a flexible, mobile, global network whose purpose is terror?

At least some of the broad outlines of an answer to global networks of terror are apparent. Strategies to prevent and contain global terrorism draw on the institutions and networks that globalization makes possible. Improved global governance, the sharing of knowledge and intelligence, forensic accounting by global financial institutions and banks, tighter coordination of international police and law enforcement and, at times, the appropriately targeted use of military force and covert operations — all are part of the long and complicated struggle. Within post-industrial societies, however, the questions are far more difficult. Terror challenges much of what defines open, multicultural, knowledge-based, democratic society.

The renewed need to provide security throws into sharp relief the new ways that states are delivering public goods. Throughout this book, we have explored the making of post-industrial society through the lens of the debates swirling around health care and public education. The language we use as we reconceive the role of the state and the way it provides these public goods tells a story of a society that is changing, with new forms of social organization and the beginnings of a smarter state that provides public goods in new ways.

As we listened to public conversations about health care and education, we heard many citizens who are now more distrustful of public authority, more confident and knowledgeable, and more protective of their rights demand enhanced accountability and greater choice among public goods. We also heard a deep ambivalence about the shape of the state: we are simultaneously turning away from the state to markets for efficiency, but we are turning back to the state again even more sharply to insist on accountability. We want to see both more and less of the state in post-industrial society. Our escape from the state, we found, was more apparent than real: as citizens who value our rights, we nevertheless continue to give the state a strong, although newly drawn, face.

The demand for security as a public good immediately confronts the language of liberties, rights, and choice. The contradictions between security and rights are sharpest because networks of terror, even when they are headquartered outside, must operate from within. The adversary is not only the other, it is also inside our societies, embedded in our rich diversity, invisible in our multicultural variety. An enemy within traditionally poses the greatest threat to liberty and to rights as the state turns inward to society to root out those hidden among us who seek to inflict terror, violence, and punishment. If there is a "war" on networks of terror, we are fighting that war on the battlefield of the societies that we have constructed and that we value.

Our language of rights is the product of a long struggle to define the appropriate balance between the individual in society and the state. As we have seen, rights language has gained force and strength in post-industrial societies as citizens have become more knowledgeable, less deferential, and more suspicious of authority. The rights revolution has empowered citizens, who have asserted their autonomy, their competency, and their right to make judgements and choices about important issues. This sense of competency, of autonomy, of independence will be put to the test as citizens demand security in the face of networks of terror. Citizens will have to choose yet again the appropriate boundaries for a state that is necessarily seeking out those living among us who are prepared to exploit our openness, our diversity, and our respect for rights in order to attack what we cherish.

These are very early days in what will be a long struggle, a struggle that will last for at least a generation. Yet the turn in the axis of public discussion is already apparent. The demand for a newly configured state, as we have seen, has often been the cloak for the political agenda of those who want the state to retreat from its managerial role in society, to pull back and slim down, and to foster efficiency through the competition that markets engender; whatever government runs, the argument goes, it runs badly. It is also the agenda of those who see the state as beholden to special interests, the creature of the politically organized and effective. Those who generally make these arguments speak with a different voice when the public good they want is security.

Those who argue loudly for limits, who support freedom from the state and the right to choice, are insisting now that the state take unto itself extensive new powers to investigate those among us who may be members of networks of terror. That same heavy-handed, bureaucratic state, which is often reviled for its invasion of liberty and its restriction of rights, is being encouraged to intervene aggressively in society to root out the enemy within. These voices have been heard before when threat looms.

This *volte face* is not restricted to those who usually speak derisively of the state as inept and inflexible, and as a threat to individual freedoms and rights. The traditional defenders of the state as the provider of choice for public goods, those who attack markets, who are prepared to accept restrictions on the right to choice to advance equity and justice, are now urging restraint on the powers that will be given to that same state. They are demanding limits on what the state can do, and asserting the primacy of rights even in the face of an enemy within. These voices, too, hearken back to earlier debates and earlier times.

Earlier debates and earlier times may not be the best guide to the dilemmas of security from terror that we confront. The familiar rhetoric of political warriors will not be adequate for the conversation that is about to begin. The conflicts among values that we face, as we saw when we looked at the public goods of health care and education, are often intractable and incommensurable, with no prospect of final resolution. And there is no more difficult conflict than that between the security of all and the rights of the individual in society. The reflexive responses, even in the urgency of crisis, have been encouraging: the almost instinctive opposition among citizens and leaders alike to the stigmatization of any of our citizens is evidence of how far we have come in a very short time. We need only think back fifty years to the Second World War to remember how badly citizens who came from the countries of adversaries were treated. Fifty years is no more than the blink of an eye in history, yet the differences in values are striking.

History shows us, however, that struggles against enemies within are not fought in the language of values. They come to life through pragmatics, as complex regulations and legal restrictions are put into place to deal with emergencies. We would do well to heed the words of a justice of the Supreme Court of the United States, who dissented from the imprisonment of a Japanese-American in 1942. Justice Robert Jackson argued that, once a judicial opinion rationalizes an emergency restriction, or even worse, rationalizes constitutional principles to show that they sanction such restrictions, "that principle then lies about like a loaded weapon ready for the hand of any authority that can bring forward a plausible claim of an urgent need."[5] It is all too easy to rush to judgement in the urgency of the moment. Yet here, too, as with other public goods, we need to keep the public conversation open. The best of our public conversations are informed not only by values, but how these values are lived in experience.

The conflict among values is real and the choices will be difficult. We will have to acknowledge as time goes on that, just as individual rights are not absolute, just as they must always be balanced against the rights of others, so we, like other post-industrial societies in different parts of the world, cannot have absolute security. Pursuit of absolute security is absolute folly; as G. K. Chesterton reminded us, the wildness of life lies in wait.

When we looked at health care and education, I argued that, as post-industrial society continues to grow and deepen, we will have to find new ways to bound possibility and openness with commitment. When the conversation shifts to the public good of security, the challenge will be to find new ways of allowing for openness in the midst of commitment. In post-industrial societies, we are not only fighting enemies "over there"; confident in our capacity as citizens to make the important choices, we are also choosing the terms of living in relative security with diversity at home. This is the challenge of constructing the public good.

NOTES

Chapter I: The Cult of Efficiency

1   Cited in Corey Robin, "The Ex-Cons: Right-Wing Thinkers Go Left!" *Lingua Franca* 11, 1 (Feb. 2001), pp. 24–33, 32.

2   Joseph Heath, *The Efficient Society: Why Canada Is as Close to Utopia as It Gets* (Toronto: Penguin, 2001), p. 84.

3   In the 1990s, governments embarked upon measures to contain public-health expenditures. Ontario and Alberta began to experiment with case-based funding formulas in restraining hospital budgets. These formulas — cost per weighted case and negotiated volumes of activity, developed with the collaboration and support of provincial hospital associations — were an attempt to reward hospitals for "efficiency."

4   *Portals and Pathways: A Review of Post-Secondary Education in Ontario, Report of the Investing in Students Task Force* (Toronto: Queen's Park, 2001) included thirty-three recommendations to increase efficiency, such as system-wide collaboration to simplify procedures for transferring

student credits and applying for student aid, as well as collaboration on future "e-learning" initiatives. See www.edu.gov.on.ca/task.

5   Ian Smilie, "NGOs and Development Assistance: A Change in Mind-set?" *Third World Quarterly* 18, 3 (1997), pp. 563–77, 566.

6   For an extension of the argument of consumerism to the home and family, see David Bosworth, "The Spirit of Capitalism 2000," *Public Interest* 138 (Winter, 2000), pp. 3–28.

7   Standing Senate Committee on Social Affairs, Science and Technology, *Final Report on Social Cohesion* (Ottawa: June 1999), available at www.parl.gc.ca/parlbus/commbus/ senate/com-e/soci-e/rep-e/repfinal/jun99-e.htm. Keith Banting makes precisely this argument in "The Internationalization of the Social Contract," in Thomas Courchene, ed., *The Nation State in a Global Information Era: Policy Challenges* (Kingston: John Deutsch Institute of Economic Research, 1999), pp. 255–85.

8   Robert Putnam, "Tuning In, Tuning Out: The Strange Disappearance of Social Capital in America," *PS: Political Science and Politics* 28 (1995), pp. 664–83.

9   Adam Smith, *An Inquiry into the Nature and Causes of the Wealth of Nations*, R. H. Campbell and A. S. Skinner, eds. (Oxford: Clarendon Press, 1975), p. 15.

10 Roland L. Meek and A. S. Skinner, "The Development of Adam Smith's Ideas on the Division of Labour," *Economic Journal* 88, 332 (1973), "Appendix A: Extracts from the 1762–3 Lecture Notes: Tuesday, April 5th, 1763," pp. 1094–116, 1100.

11 Adam Smith, in his *Theory of Moral Sentiments*, D. D. Raphael and A. L. Macfie, eds. (Oxford: Clarendon Press, 1976), argues that "human sympathy" is the basis

for social cohesion and an important corrective to an unhindered free market.

12 Smith, *Wealth of Nations*, pp. 26–27.

13 Plato, *Republic*, A. D. Linsay, ed. (London: Dent, 1976), p. 49.

14 S. Todd Lowry, *The Archaeology of Economic Ideas: The Classical Greek Tradition* (Durham, NC: Duke University Press, 1987), p. 108.

15 Lewis Mumford, *The Pentagon of Power: The Myth of the Machine*, vol. 2 (New York: Harcourt Brace Jovanovich, 1970).

16 Ibid, p. 173.

17 Anson Rabinbach, *The Human Motor: Energy, Fatigue, and the Origins of Modernity* (New York: Basic Books), p. 127.

18 Cited in ibid.

19 Heath, *Efficient Society*, p. 12.

20 Frederick Winslow Taylor, *The Principles of Scientific Management* (1911; reprint, New York: Harper and Bros., 1947).

21 Andrew Sharpe, "Determinants of Trends in Living Standards in Canada and the United States, 1989–2000," *International Productivity Monitor*, 2 (Spring 2001), pp. 3–10.

22 There are different approaches, interpretations, and statistical requirements of productivity measures, and little consensus among experts on appropriate concepts and measures. See Paul Schreyer, "The OECD Productivity Manual: A Guide to the Measurement of Industry-Level and Aggregate Productivity," *International Productivity Monitor*, 2 (Spring 2001), pp. 37–51.

23 Rabinbach, *Human Motor*, p. 129.

24 James Allen Smith, *The Idea Brokers* (New York: The Free Press, 1991), p. 48.

25 William H. Allen, *Efficient Democracy* (New York: Dodd, Mead and Co., 1907, 1912), p. 281.

26 This account of municipal reform draws on Smith, *Idea Brokers*, p. 47ff.

27 The political agenda of the reformers who used the language of efficiency was to develop and insulate the power of emerging metropolitan commercial and technical elites from the sustained pressures of machine politics. Martin J. Schiesl, *The Politics of Efficiency: Municipal Administration and Reform in America, 1800–1920* (Berkeley: University of California Press, 1977), p. 192.

28 As Theodore Lowi and Edward J. Harpham observe: "Although Weberian state theory does not rely on human perfectibility, it has come close to an ideology of institutional perfectibility." See "Political Theory and Public Policy," in Kristen R. Monroe, ed., *Contemporary Empirical Political Theory* (Berkeley: University of California Press, 1997), pp. 249–78, 264.

29 Deborah Stone, *Policy Paradox and Political Reason* (New York: HarperCollins, 1988), pp. 13, 53.

30 Heath, *Efficient Society*, pp. 18–21.

31 Later utilitarians considered the consequences of action not only on the happiness of the greatest number of members of the community currently living, but on future generations as well. Henry Sidgwick, writing in the late nineteenth century, claimed a "general — if not universal — assent for the principle that the true standard and criterion by which right legislation is to be distinguished from wrong is conducive to the general good or 'welfare.' And probably the majority of persons would agree to interpret the 'good' or 'welfare' of the community to mean, in the last analysis, the happiness of the individual human

beings who compose the community; provided that we take into account not only the human beings who are actually living but those who are to live hereafter." Sidgwick, *The Elements of Politics* (London: Macmillan, 1891), p. 34, cited in John Morrow, *History of Political Thought: A Thematic Introduction* (London: Macmillan, 1998), p. 120. Productive efficiency that increases pollution for future generations would then not be considered "efficient."

32 Amartya K. Sen, "Rational Fools: A Critique of the Behavioural Foundations of Economic Theory," *Philosophy and Public Affairs* 6, 4 (1977), pp. 317–44.

33 Richard Ned Lebow and Janice Gross Stein, *We All Lost the Cold War* (Princeton NJ: Princeton University Press, 1991), pp. 294–95.

34 Jeremy Bentham, *Principles of Morals and Legislation*, J. H. Burns and H. L. A. Hart, eds. (Oxford: Clarendon Press, 1996), pp. 11–15.

35 Bentham, *A Fragment on Government and an Introduction to Principles of Morals and Legislation*, Wilfred Harrison, ed. (Oxford: Blackwell, 1967), p. 125.

36 Ibid, p. 127.

37 Vilfredo Pareto, *Manual of Political Economy*, Ann S. Schwier and Alfred N. Page, trans. (New York: A. M. Kelley, 1971), ch. 6, sec. 33, p. 261ff.

38 Axel van den Berg, "Politics versus Markets: A Note on the Uses of Double Standards" (paper presented to Reinventing Society in a Changing Global Economy Conference, University of Toronto, Toronto, March 8–9, 2001), p. 1. I draw heavily on his argument in the paragraphs that follow, and in the analysis of states and markets in the section that follows.

39 Ibid.

40   Albert O. Hirschman, *Rival Views of Market Society and Other Recent Essays* (New York: Viking, 1986), p. 107.

41   Stephen Holmes, "The Secret History of Self-Interest," in Jane J. Mansbridge, ed., *Beyond Self-Interest* (Chicago: University of Chicago Press, 1990), pp. 267–86.

42   Kristen R. Monroe, "Human Nature, Identity, and Politics," in *Contemporary Empirical Political Theory*, pp. 279–306, 282. There is robust evidence from contemporary research in psychology that demonstrates people rarely conform to this ideal of rational, efficient choice when they make decisions.

43   Heath, *Efficient Society*, p. 201.

44   Hayek, unlike Smith and Friedman, built his defence of the free market on a radical subjectivity. He argued that economic value — the value of an asset or a resource — is wholly a product of the preferences or values of individuals, and not of any of its objective properties. It was not capital or labour that gave value to goods, but preferences alone. Rational utility maximization was also not the most compelling explanation of markets. Beneath the patina of rationality was inchoate thinking that was inaccessible in either theoretical or technical terms. It was the particular genius of the market to harness these inchoate longings to economic activity. See John Gray, *Hayek on Liberty* (Oxford: Blackwell, 1984) and Robin, "The Ex-Cons."

45   Smith, *Theory of Moral Sentiments*, pp. 380–81, cited by van den Berg, "Politics versus Markets," p. 6. Van den Berg eloquently develops this argument.

46   Holmes, "Secret History," pp. 285–86.

47   Public choice scholarship, as it is known, has formalized and generalized the argument that government regulation serves as a cloak for sectional interests. See Anthony

Downs, *An Economic Theory of Democracy* (New York: Harper and Row, 1957); Gordon Tullock, *Private Wants, Public Means: An Economic Analysis of the Desirable Scope of Government* (New York: Basic Books, 1970); James M. Buchanan and Robert D. Tollison, eds., *Theory of Public Choice: Political Application of Economics* (Ann Arbor: University of Michigan Press, 1972); and Andrei Shleifer and Robert Vishny, *The Grabbing Hand: Government Pathologies and Their Cures* (Cambridge, MA: Harvard University Press, 1998).

48 Robert Mundell, lecture at the University of Toronto, March 15, 2001.

49 Douglass North, *Structure and Change in Economic History* (New York: Norton, 1981).

50 Smith, *Wealth of Nations*, p. 232.

51 Axel van den Berg and Joseph Smucker, eds., *The Sociology of Labour Markets: Efficiency, Equity, Security* (Toronto: Prentice-Hall Canada, 1997).

52 Ibid, p. 196.

53 Jeremy Bentham, *Economic Writings*, vol.3, W. Stark, ed. (London: Allen and Unwin, 1954), pp. 257–58.

54 Van den Berg, "Politics versus Markets," p. 12.

Chapter II: Efficiency and Accountability in the Post-industrial Age

1 John O'Neill, *The Poverty of Postmodernism* (New York: Routledge, 1995), p. 111.

2 Heath, *Efficient Society*, p. xviii.

3 Francis Fukuyama, *The End of History and the Last Man* (New York: Avon, 1992).

4 Critics of globalization, drawing on the Gramscian tradition, examine the ideological processes that have

displaced traditional embedded liberalism and enshrined market liberalism, deregulation, and privatization. They treat globalization as a "hegemonic discourse" that alters ideas and expectations about the role of the state. See Philip Cerny, "Globalization and Other Stories: The Search for a New Paradigm for International Relations," *International Journal* 51, 4 (1996), pp. 617–37. For an analysis of these processes in Canada, see H. W. Arthurs, "Globalization of the Mind: Canadian Elites and the Restructuring of Legal Fields," *Canadian Journal of Law and Society* 12, 2 (1997), pp. 219-46. But see also Bob Rae's argument that globalization is often used as a convenient excuse for already existing preferences for a restricted state. Bob Rae, *The Three Questions: Prosperity and the Public Good* (Toronto: Viking, 1998).

5　　Countervailing tendencies also exist: knowledge can be a source of competitive advantage, and the current state-led attempt to strengthen the international regime protecting intellectual property rights seeks to reterritorialize knowledge and convert it into a private good.

6　　For an analysis of knowledge networks, see Janice Gross Stein, Richard Stren, Joy Fitzgibbon, and Melissa MacLean, *Networks of Knowledge: Collaborative Innovations in International Learning* (Toronto: University of Toronto Press, 2001).

7　　Jeffrey Sachs, "International Economics: Unlocking the Mysteries of Globalization," *Foreign Policy* 110 (1998), pp. 97–111.

8　　Mark Zacher, "The Global Economy and the International Political Order," in Thomas Courchene, ed., *The Nation-state in a Global/Information Era: Policy Challenges* (Kingston: John Deutsch Institute for Economic Research,

1999), pp. 67–95. See also Michael T. Greven and Louis W. Pauly, eds., *Democracy Beyond the State? The European Dilemma and the Emerging Global Order* (Latham, MD: Rowman and Littlefield, 2000); and David Held, *Democracy and the Global Order: From the Modern State to Cosmopolitan Governance* (Stanford, CA: Stanford University Press, 1995).

9   Tom J. Courchene and John N. McDougall, "The Contest for Future Constitutional Options," in Ronald B. Watts and Douglas M. Brown, eds., *Options for a New Canada* (Toronto: University of Toronto Press, 1991), pp. 33–51.

10   For a sceptical view, see Louis Pauly, *Who Elected the Bankers? Surveillance and Control in the World Economy* (Ithaca, NY: Cornell University Press, 1997).

11   Kenici Ohmae, in *The End of the Nation-state* (New York: Free Press, 1995), p. 5, argues: "Traditional nation-states have become unnatural, even impossible, business units in a global economy." Susan Strange made a similar argument: "The impersonal forces of world markets . . . are now more powerful than the states to whom ultimate political authority over society and economy is supposed to belong. . . . The declining authority of states is reflected in a growing diffusion of authority to other institutions and associations, and to local and regional bodies." Strange, *The Retreat of the State: The Diffusion of Power in the World Economy* (Cambridge: Cambridge University Press, 1996), p. 4.

12   Manuel Castells, *The Rise of the Network Society* (Oxford: Blackwell, 1990) and John Ruggie, *Winning the Peace: America and World Order in the New Era* (New York: Columbia University Press, 1996).

13   Yale Ferguson and Richard Mansbach, *Polities: Authority,*

Identities, and Change (Columbia, SC: University of South Carolina Press, 1996).

14 Borders matter as well. In 1996, the typical Canadian province traded twelve times as much with another Canadian province as it did with a state in the U.S. of similar size and distance. There are still significant border effects within the European Union, the most densely integrated economy, for goods, services, and capital. The markets for domestic goods are still much tighter than international markets. John Helliwell, *Globalization: Myths, Facts, and Consequences* (Toronto: C. D. Howe, 2000), pp. 3ff.

15 Geoffrey Garrett, "Global Markets and National Politics: Collision Course or Virtuous Circle," *International Organization* 52, 4 (1998), 787–824. See also Geoffrey Garrett and Peter Lange, "Internationalization, Institutions, and Political Change," in Helen Milner and Robert Keohane, eds., *Internationalization and Domestic Politics* (Cambridge: Cambridge University Press, 1996), pp. 48–75, and A. Hurrell and N. Woods, "Globalization and Inequality," *Millennium* 24, 3 (1995), pp. 447–70. David Held argues that the state has the capacity to reconstitute and transform itself to respond to the more active global agenda. Held, *Global Transformations* (Stanford, CA: Stanford University Press, 1999), p. 436.

16 Dani Rodrik, "Why Do More Open Economies Have Bigger Governments?" *Journal of Political Economy* (forthcoming 2001).

17 Paul Abramson and Ronald Inglehart, *Value Change in Global Perspective* (Ann Arbor, MI: University of Michigan Press, 1995).

18 Neil Nevitte, "Value Change and Reorientations in

Citizen-State Relations," *Canadian Public Policy* 26 (2000), pp. 73–94.

19 Daniel Bell, *The Cultural Contradictions of Capitalism* (New York: Basic Books, 1976) and *The Coming of Post-industrial Society* (New York: Basic Books, 1973), pp. 148–49; and Peter Ester, Leok Halman, and Ruud de Moor, "Value Shift in Western Societies," in Ester, Halman, and de Moor, eds., *Value Change in Europe and North America* (Tilburg, Neth.: Tilburg University Press, 1993), pp. 1–20.

20 Ronald Inglehart, *Modernization and Postmodernization: Cultural, Economic, and Political Change in 43 Societies* (Princeton, NJ: Princeton University Press, 1997).

21 Interview with Antonio Negri in Mark Leonard, "The Left Should Love Globalization," *New Statesman*, May 28, 2001, p. 37. See also Antonio Negri and Michael Hardt, *Empire* (Cambridge, MA: Harvard University Press, 2000).

22 Peter Warrian, "From Industrywide Bargaining to Individuation: Changing Social Values of Local Union Leaders" (unpublished paper, Toronto, April 2001). Warrian draws on data gathered by the Environics Research Group in the winter and spring of 1999. See also Peter Warrian, *Hard Bargain: Transforming Public-Sector Labour-Management Relations* (Toronto: McGilligan Books, 1996).

23 Michael Ignatieff, *The Rights Revolution* (Toronto: Anansi, 2000), p. 1.

24 Ibid, p. 36.

25 Amartya K. Sen, *Development As Freedom* (New York: Knopf, 1999), pp. xi, xii; and *Poverty and Famines: An Essay on Entitlement and Deprivation* (Oxford: Clarendon Press, 1982).

26 Robert Sheppard, "We Are Canadian," *Maclean's* 113/114, 52/1 (Dec. 25, 2000/Jan. 1, 2001), p. 30.

27 Robert Marshall, "Paying the Price," *Maclean's* 113/114, 52/1 (Dec. 25, 2000/Jan. 1, 2001), p. 50.

28 Samuel Barnes et al., *Political Action: Mass Participation in Five Western Democracies* (Beverly Hills: Sage Publications, 1979).

29 Nevitte, "Value Change and Reorientations," p. 77.

30 Warrian, "From Industrywide Bargaining to Individuation."

31 M. Alvin and M. Sverke, "Do New Generations Imply the End of Solidarity? Swedish Unionism in the Era of Individualization," *Economics and Industrial Democracy* 21, 1 (2000), pp. 71–95.

32 Inglehart, *Modernization and Post-Modernization*, pp. 260–61.

33 Michael Barzelay, *Breaking through Bureaucracy: A New Vision for Managing in Government* (Berkeley: University of California Press, 1992).

34 Peter Senge, *The Fifth Discipline: The Art and Practice of the Learning Organization* (New York: Doubleday, 1990).

35 Lloyd A. Blanchard, Charles C. Hinnant, and Wilson Wong, "Market-Based Reforms: Toward a Social Subcontract?" *Administration and Society* 30, 5 (1998), pp. 483–512.

36 William Coleman, "The Project on Trends: An Introduction," *Canadian Public Policy* 26 (2000), pp. 1–14.

37 Heath, *Efficient Society*, pp. xviii, 7.

38 Aaron Wildavsky, *Speaking Truth to Power: The Art and Craft of Policy Analysis* (Boston: Little Brown, 1979), p. 131.

39 Heath recognizes this argument in other parts of his analysis. "Instead of creating more leisure time so that we can concentrate on the things that really matter to us,

efficiency seems to be becoming an end in itself. People no longer seek efficiency in order to achieve their other goals; they pursue it for their own sake." *Efficient Society*, p. 225.

40 Allan R. Gregg, "A Shifting Landscape," *Maclean's* 113/114, 52/1 (Dec. 25, 2000/Jan. 1. 2001), p. 35.

41 The technical definition of cost-effectiveness is the maximum possible output obtained from a given quantity of inputs, or a given output achieved with minimum inputs. The sector, or the facility, is then operating at the production possibility frontier.

42 These questions about the allocation of resources across a sector that delivers public goods speak to what economists call maximum social welfare. Social welfare is the aggregation of subjective individual welfare, except under very specific conditions when markets fail. Social welfare means something quite different to those who worry about equity or justice. Here, welfare is designed for society as a whole, and it requires external standards rather than internal measures to evaluate effectiveness. The difference is not trivial. For discussion of the different meanings of equity, see Deborah Stone, *Policy Paradox and Political Reason* (New York: Harper Collins, 1988), pp. 30–48.

43 Arthur Okun, *Equality and Efficiency: The Big Trade-Off* (Washington, D.C.: Brookings Institution, 1975).

44 Albert O. Hirschman, *Exit, Voice, and Loyalty: Responses to Decline in Firms, Organizations, and States* (Cambridge, MA: Harvard University Press, 1970).

45 There is some evidence that private contractors see reduced information requirements in comparison to what public providers must supply as one of the efficiency gains. Richard Mulgan, "The Processes of Public

Accountability," *Australian Journal of Public Administration* 56, 1 (March 1997), pp. 25–36.

46   Ignatieff, *The Rights Revolution*, p. 2.

Chapter III: Efficiency and Choice: Public Education and Health Care

1   Margaret Wente, "The Case for School Choice: Something for Lefties and Righties," *Globe and Mail*, April 17, 2001, p. A19.

2   William Thorsell, "Stockwell Agonistes and the New Political Math," *Globe and Mail*, July 9, 2001, p. A13.

3   Gina Feldberg and Robert Vipond, "The Virus of Consumerism," in Daniel Drache and Terry Sullivan, eds., *Market Limits in Health Reform: Public Success, Private Failure* (London: Routledge, 1999), pp. 48–64.

4   Ken Pole, "Canadians Concerned about the Efficiency and Accountability of Care," *The Medical Post* 37, 9 (Mar. 6, 2001). There is a curious paradox here: although Canadians are more likely than Australians, New Zealanders, Britons, or Americans to rate the medical care they received in the past twelve months as excellent, they worry that the health-care system is seriously under pressure now, and that it will be even less able to meet their needs in the future. R. J. Blendon et al., "The Cost of Health System Change: Public Discontent in Five Nations," *Health Affairs* 18, 3 (May–June 1999), pp. 206–16. Eighty percent of Canadians believe that the system is in crisis. Sheppard, "We Are Canadian," p. 28, and Marshall, "Paying the Price," pp. 48–50; John Schofield, "Saving Our Schools," *Maclean's* (May 14, 2000), pp. 22–29, and Gregg, "A Shifting Landscape," p. 34.

5 A very slim majority of Canadians support user fees either to curb "inappropriate" use or to generate additional funds, and are not opposed to a two-tier medical system if — and this is an important if — the publicly funded system is unable to provide necessary services. Marshall, "Paying the Price." Only 15 percent of Canadians are willing to pay higher taxes, and 70 percent said there is room for cutting costs within the system. PricewaterhouseCoopers conducted the survey. Jill Mahoney, "Private Health Care OK, with Conditions, Poll Finds," *Globe and Mail*, July 3, 2001, p. A4.

6 Canada has a reasonably efficient health care system. It spends about 9 percent of its gross domestic product on health care, less than France, Switzerland, Germany, and the United States. In 1998, Canada ranked fifth in total expenditure on health per capita among the twenty-two members of the Organization for Economic Cooperation and Development. Canadian Institute for Health Information, *Health Care in Canada* (Ottawa: Statistics Canada, 2001), p. 72. That Canada spends less on health care than some other post-industrial societies will not make the health-care system efficient if the care Canadians receive is less effective. Yet Canada's infant mortality rate is lower than that of the United States, and its life expectancy is longer. In a comparison of the health profiles of post-industrial societies that taps measures more directly related to health care, Canada ranked first, ahead of Norway, Japan, Sweden, the United Kingdom, and the United States.

7 Experts discount the dismal results to some degree because students knew that the test did not count.

8 The cry of alarm is hardly unique to Ontario. Scores from

the Canadian Test of Basic Skills show a long-term decline in the performance of grade-eight students, especially in language skills. In 1989, Statistics Canada found that more than a quarter of Canadians from the ages of sixteen to twenty-four lacked basic "everyday" reading skills, and 44 percent were below that standard in numeracy. In international tests of knowledge of mathematics and science, ten-year-old Canadians compare well to others in post-industrial societies; by fourteen, the relative position of Canadian students begins to slip, and by the end of high school, Canadian students are well below the average level. Economic Council of Canada, *A Lot to Learn: Education and Training in Canada* (Ottawa: Minister of Supply and Services, 1992).

9   Ronald Manzer, *Public Schools and Political Ideas: Canadian Educational Policy in Historical Perspective* (Toronto: University of Toronto Press, 1994), p. 256.

10   Murray Campbell, "For Most Canadians, Our History is a Mystery," *Globe and Mail*, June 30, 2001, pp. A1, A7.

11   After inflation, spending on health care grew by 4.4 percent in 1999 and another 4.9 percent in 2000. In Ontario, provincial spending has risen from 38 percent to 43 percent of the government's budget, and some project that spending will grow to 60 percent in the next five years if the health-care system is not changed. These numbers are disputed because what the government has included in government spending has varied over time. The government of Quebec spends 40 percent of its budget on health care.

12   In Saskatchewan, spending grew by 7 percent in 1999 and 3.1 percent in 2000. If no new programs and no additional personnel are added to the health-care system in

Saskatchewan, if the system stays the way it is and takes on no new challenges, the health budget will still have to grow by 6.5 percent a year. Government revenues to fund health care are projected to grow at no more than 3 percent a year. *Caring for Medicare: Sustaining a Quality System* (Saskatoon: Commission on Medicare, April 2001), pp. 71, 75. Available at www.medicare-commission.com/reports.htm.

13 Cam Donaldson, Gillian Currie, and Craig Milton, *Integrating Canada's Dis-Integrated Health Care System* (Toronto: C. D. Howe Institute, 2001), p. 20.

14 The evidence of the impact of socio-economic status on educational achievement is consistent and solid. The pioneering study is James S. Coleman et al., *Equality of Educational Opportunity* (Washington, D.C.: Department of Health, Education, and Welfare, 1966). See also Eric Hanushek, "The Economics of Schooling: Production and Efficiency in Public Schools," *Journal of Economic Literature* 24, 3 (Sept., 1986), pp. 1141–77, and John Chubb and Terry Moe, *Politics, Markets, and America's Schools* (Washington, D.C.: Brookings Institution, 1990), p. 101.

15 Francine Dube, "I Love This School," *National Post*, April 23, 2001, p. A15.

16 For a description of the centralized system of public education as a "factory," see Bruce J. Fuller, ed., *Inside Charter Schools: The Paradox of Radical Decentralization* (Cambridge, MA: Harvard University Press, 2000).

17 David B. Tyack, *The One Best System: A History of American Urban Education* (Cambridge, MA: Harvard University Press, 1974). The "one best system" emerged from a political process of pulling and hauling that privileged the middle class and the new educational professionals who

ran the system. For Canada, see Manzer, *Public Schools and Political Ideas*.

18 Physician fees declined by 18 percent in Canada and rose by 22 percent in the United States, and office expenses were 36 percent of gross billings in Canada and 48 percent in the United States. General Accounting Office, *Canadian Health Insurance: Lessons for the United States*, Report to the Chairman, Committee on Government Operations, House of Representatives (Washington, D.C.: United States GAO, 1991), pp. 5, 35, cited in Carolyn Tuohy, *Accidental Logics: The Dynamics of Change in the Health Care Arena in the United States, Britain, and Canada* (New York: Oxford University Press, 1999), p. 206.

19 Raisa Deber, *Getting What We Pay For: Myths and Realities about Financing Canada's Health Care System* (paper prepared for the National Dialogue on Health Reform, April 11, 2000).

20 Institute for Research on Public Policy (IRPP), *IRPP Task Force on Health Policy: Recommendations to First Ministers* (Montreal: IRPP, 2000), p. 5.

21 Thomas Paine, *Rights of Man*, in Michael Foot and Isaac Kramnick, eds., *Thomas Paine Reader* (New York: Penguin Books, 1987), pp. 201–364, 335.

22 Milton Friedman, "The Role of Government in Education," in Robert A. Solow, ed., *Economics and the Public Interest* (New Brunswick, NJ: Rutgers Press, 1955), pp. 123–44; and Michael Trebilcock, Ron Daniels, and Malcolm Thorburn, "Government by Voucher," *Boston University Law Review* 80 (2000), pp. 205–32.

23 The term "monopoly" is not a wholly accurate description of the Canadian educational market. In Canada, approximately 5 percent of students attend private schools, half as

many as do in the United States, largely because Ontario and Quebec provide funding for some religious schools, Alberta and Saskatchewan fund Roman Catholic schools, and British Columbia, Quebec, and Alberta provide up to 60 percent of the per pupil funding to private schools. See www.statscan.ca/english/Pgdb/People/Education/educo1.htm and www.direct.ca/fisa/fisc/funding.htm.

24 Chubb and Moe, *Politics, Markets, and America's Schools*, p. 183. See www.statscan.ca/english/Pgdb/People/Education/educo1.htm and www.direct.ca/fisa/fisc/funding.htm.

25 There are clear differences in Canada in the quality of education provided to children from affluent and low-income families, largely because better public schools are usually located in wealthier neighbourhoods. John H. Bishop, "Privatizing Education: Lessons from Canada and Europe," in C. Eugene Steuerle, Van Doorn Ooms, George Peterson, and Robert Reischauer, eds., *Vouchers and the Provision of Public Services* (Washington: Brookings Institution, 2000), pp. 291–335, 292.

26 John F. Witte, *The Market Approach to Education: An Analysis of America's First Voucher Program* (Princeton, NJ: Princeton University Press, 2000), p. 42.

27 Milwaukee Public School cost per student was $3,469, while the cost per voucher student was $4,373, or 20 percent higher. John Witte, who was officially appointed to evaluate the Milwaukee voucher program, concluded that there is little evidence for an efficiency argument for voucher schools. Witte, *Market Approach to Education*, p. 106.

28 Ibid, pp. 112–51. Paul Peterson, a prominent proponent of voucher programs, ferociously attacked Witte's results

and claimed that children who stayed in the voucher program for four years outperformed a control group of students in math, but not in reading. Jay Greene, Paul Peterson, and J. Du, "Effectiveness of School Choice: The Milwaukee Experiment," Department of Government, Harvard University, 1997, unpublished report. However, very few children stayed for four years. A third analysis by Cecilia Rouse found an improvement of 1.5 to 2.3 percentile points for voucher students in math and no effect on reading. Cecilia Rouse, "Private School Vouchers and Student Achievement: An Evaluation of the Milwaukee Parental Choice Program," *Quarterly Journal of Economics* 113, 2 (May 1998), pp. 553–602.

29 The issue is confused in public debate with public funding for religious schools. The principle of equality of funding to religious schools has the support of the United Nations Human Rights Commission, which in 1999 urged Ontario to extend funding to all religious schools, not just to Roman Catholic schools. The Sullivan Royal Commission in British Columbia went further in its report in 1998 in endorsing provincial funding to private schools: "Such aid we believe to be a normal tangible manifestation of the freedom of thought, belief, opinion, and expression guaranteed by the Charter of Rights and Freedoms." Cited by Daniel Girard, "Schoolhouse Dues: Public Cash for Private Education Has a Long History Out West," *Toronto Star*, May 13, 2001, p. A9. Their opinions do not, however, necessarily imply voucher programs; a system of grants would meet the requirement as well. Quebec, Manitoba, Alberta, Saskatchewan, and British Columbia all fund religious schools, but very differently: they give per student grants to the schools directly. The Ontario program would

allow parents who send their children to a religious school to receive the tax credit, but all private schools, not only religious schools, are eligible.

30 Claudia R. Hepburn, ed., *Can the Markets Save Our Schools?* (Vancouver: Fraser Institute, 2001), cited by Julie Smyth, "Tax Credit May Aid All Schools," *National Post*, June 21, 2001, p. A9.

31 Earl Manners, "Budget Spells Two-Tier Education," *Toronto Star*, May 11, 2001, p. A21. The direct savings to the government, however, are clear: it costs the government about $7,500 for every student who stays in the public system; for every student who leaves, the government saves $4,000. This is cost-cutting masked as efficiency. Savings are realized by creating incentives for students to leave the public system.

32 I am indebted to Ron Manzer for this point. Personal communication, May 29, 2001.

33 Legally, physicians in Canada can opt out of medicare and bill privately, but very few physicians have done so. The most accurate way to describe the Canadian system is as a mixed publicly and privately financed system across the continuum of health care, that is delivered through private medical providers whose fees are negotiated, not-for-profit institutions that provide acute care and are funded directly by provincial governments, and private providers in the regulated health professions who charge their patients as they see fit for services that are not considered medically necessary. Few Canadians would recognize this longer, but more accurate, description of their health-care system: the word "private" appears far more often than Canadians would generally expect.

34 David Gratzer, *Code Blue: Reviving Canada's Health Care System* (Toronto: ECW Press, 1999), p. 181.

35 Deber, *We Get What We Pay For*, p. 40, and "Interview of Robert Evans," The Atkinson Letter, *Medicare in Crisis: Myths and Realities* (Toronto: The Atkinson Foundation, November 29, 1996).

36 Deber, *We Get What We Pay For*, p. 10, and "Interview of Robert Evans," *Medicare in Crisis.*

37 Within the United Kingdom, regions with high levels of private insurance were likely to have the largest waiting lists. In Manitoba, physicians were allowed to perform cataract surgery on a private basis, although they were subsidized by medicare. Analysis of the waiting times tells an interesting story: they were shortest — four weeks — for those using the privately provided services; longer — ten weeks — for those using surgeons who worked only in the public sector; and longest — twenty-three weeks — for publicly financed surgery performed by those who practised in both sectors. Carolyn DeCoster, K. C. Carriere, Sandra Peterson, Randy Wald, and Leonard MacWilliam, *Surgical Waiting Times in Manitoba* (Winnipeg: Manitoba Centre for Health Policy and Evaluation, 1998). Available at www.umanitoba.ca/centres/mchpe/wait.htm. All the evidence on waiting lists and times is drawn from Carolyn Tuohy, Colleen Flood, and Mark Stabile, "How Does Private Finance Affect Public Health Care Systems?" (University of Toronto working paper, 2001), p. 14.

38 Gratzer, *Code Blue*, p. 190ff; William McArthur, Cynthia Ramsay, and Michael Walker, eds., *Healthy Incentives: Canadian Health Reform in an International Context* (Vancouver: Fraser Institute, 1996); J. Gardner, "Medical

Savings Accounts Make Waves," *Modern Healthcare* 25, 9 (1995), pp. 57–62; and Fred McMahon, "Public Funding with Market Dynamics," *Policy Options* 21, 4 (May 2000), pp. 9–11.

39 If people choose to spend more than the average weighted patient in any given year, they pay privately until they reach the level where the catastrophic insurance begins. If they spend less, they can either save the money for the following year or withdraw the funds to spend for other purposes.

40 The plan in Singapore limits coverage to $70,000 Singapore dollars annually, with lifetime coverage of $200,000.

41 W. Hsiao, "Medical Savings Accounts: Lessons from Singapore," *Health Affairs* 14, 2 (1995), pp. 260–66, and T. A. Massaro and Y. Wong, "Positive Experience with Medical Savings Accounts in Singapore," *Health Affairs* 14, 2 (1995), pp. 267–72, both cited in Donaldson, Currie, and Mitton, *Integrating Canada's Dis-Integrated Health Care System*, p. 18; and Raisa Deber, "Medical Savings Accounts: A Fine Idea Unless You're Sick," *Health Policy Forum* (Spring 1999), pp. 4–5.

42 There are other difficulties. It is not easy to determine the amount of a health-care voucher. If the payment were uniform, inevitable differences across regions in the prices set by health-care providers and the supply of services would have serious consequences for the value of vouchers in different parts of a province. The supply of health-care services is much greater in Regina, for example, than it is in Moose Jaw. Smaller communities are unlikely to offer many choices to patients in the specialized and acute-care sectors, so hospitals might well be in a monopoly position

and be able to charge prices that are far higher than those in larger centres, where there would be competition. Many services and institutions that meet the needs of relatively specialized groups would find it very difficult to survive. Specialists in smaller communities would simply not attract enough "business," and small communities could lose much of their specialized care. Hospitals that specialize and provide advanced research and training — the Hospital for Sick Children in Toronto is a good example — would face similar kinds of difficulties. And it is not clear how health and medical research and information would be funded. A public voucher system that works entirely in the marketplace would find it difficult to finance those public goods and services that serve special needs or the broad collective good in a longer time frame. Most proponents of medical savings accounts make no provision for these kinds of challenges.

43 Gov. Thomas Thompson, State of the State Address (Madison, Wisconsin, January 1995), cited by Witte, *Market Approach to Education*, p. 163.

44 In the United States, many state governments require charter schools to participate in statewide testing programs, publish student test scores, and submit annual financial statements. This is also the case in Alberta, where charter schools also must be non-denominational, and cannot charge tuition fees, be for-profit, or discriminate in student admission.

45 Chester E. Finn, Jr., Bruno V. Manno, and Gregg Vanourek, *Charter Schools in Action: Renewing Public Education* (Princeton, NJ: Princeton University Press, 2000), p. 71.

46 Paul Berman et al., *The State of Charter Schools 2000: Fourth-Year Report* (Washington, D.C.: U.S. Department of

Education, Office of Educational Research and Development, 2000). In Alberta, parent satisfaction levels are generally high, and 82 percent of parents intend to keep their children in the schools. Lynn Bosetti et al., *Canadian Charter Schools at the Crossroads: Executive Summary* (Kelowna, BC: Society for the Advancement of Excellence in Education, 2000). In a survey of parents with children in charter schools, more than 60 percent said they preferred the charter schools to the public schools their children had previously attended. Finn, Manno, and Vanourek, *Charter Schools in Action.*

47   Joanne Izu et al., *Cross-Site Report: An Evaluation of Charter Schools in Los Angeles Unified School District* (San Francisco: WestEd, 1998), and Bosetti et al., *Canadian Charter Schools at the Crossroads.*

48   Bruce Fuller, "Breaking Away or Pulling Together? Making Decentralization Work," in Fuller, *Inside Charter Schools*, pp. 230–54, 231.

49   Ibid, p. 34.

50   David Bositis has conducted parallel annual surveys of African Americans and the rest of the population on education issues since 1996. He finds support for vouchers is strongest among African Americans under fifty years old, and he expects support to grow over time. "School Vouchers Along the Color Line," *New York Times*, August 15, 2001, p. A27.

51   David Matthews, "Public Government/Public Schools," *National Civic Review* 85, 3 (Fall 1996), pp. 14-22, 15.

52   Finn, Manno, and Vanourek, *Charter Schools in Action*, pp. 223–25, and Francis Fukuyama, *Trust: The Social Virtues and the Creation of Prosperity* (New York: Free Press, 1995), p. 226.

53 Mark Schneider, "Institutional Arrangements and the Creation of Social Capital: The Effects of Public School Choice," *American Political Science Review* 91, 1 (March 1997), pp. 82–93.

54 An independent assessment of charter schools in Arizona, where one in four charters nationally is located, found a widespread pattern of racial separation. Gene V. Glass, *Education Policy Analysis Archives* 7, 1 (1999), cited by Fuller, *Inside Charter Schools*, p. 37.

55 Ibid.

56 Joseph Kahne, "Democratic Communities, Equity, and Excellence: A Deweyan Reframing of Educational Policy Analysis," *Educational Evaluation and Policy Analysis* 3, 16 (Fall 1994), pp. 233–48.

57   James W. Ceasar and Patrick J. McGuinn, "Civic Education Reconsidered," *The Public Interest* 133 (Fall 1998), pp. 84–103, 103.

58 Fuller makes this argument eloquently. See Fuller, *Inside Charter Schools*, pp. 24, 28.

59 Lynn Bosetti, "Alberta Charter Schools: Paradox and Promises," *Alberta Journal of Educational Research* 66, 2 (Summer 2000), pp. 179–90.

60 M. Buechler, *Charter Schools: Legislation and Results After Four Years* (Bloomington, IN: Indiana Education Policy Centre, 1995), cited in Lynn Bosetti, "The Dark Promise of Charter Schools," *Policy Options* 19, 6 (July–Aug. 1998), pp. 63–67, 64.

61 Finn, Manno, and Vanourek, *Charter Schools in Action*, p. 21.

62 Fuller, *Inside Charter Schools*, p. 237.

63 Monique Jérôme-Forget, Joseph White, and Joshua M. Wiener, eds., *Health Care Reform through Internal Markets:*

Experience and Proposals (Montreal: Institute for Research on Public Policy, 1995), pp. 7–16, 8.

64 Richard B. Saltman, "The Role of Competitive Incentives in Recent Reforms of Northern European Health Systems," in ibid, pp. 75–94.

65 In Great Britain, there was a political as well as an economic agenda in the changes that led to the creation of markets within the public system and the purchaser-provider split in the 1990s. These markets would buffer political leaders; restructuring of the health-care sector could be explained as the result of competition. Tuohy, *Accidental Logics*, p. 169.

66 This is not the case in Sweden, where patients can choose and the money follows the patient. Saltman, "Recent Reforms of Northern European Health Systems," p. 83.

67 Physicians continued to be paid by a mixture of salary, fee-for-service, and capitation.

68 Donaldson, Currie, and Milton, *Integrating Canada's Dis-Integrated Health Care System*, p. 14.

69 Referrals to specialists did not drop in England, but they did in Scotland for certain groups. Not much can be made of these results.

70 Market elements, through the logic of the British public health system, were absorbed into existing hierarchical and professional networks. Tuohy, *Accidental Logics*, p. 199.

71 R. Klein and J. Dixon, "Cash Bonanza for NHS: The Price Is Centralization," *British Medical Journal* 320, 7239 (2000), pp. 883–84, 883.

72 R. Paul Shaw, *New Trends in Public-Sector Management in Health: Applications in Developed and Developing Countries* (Washington, D.C.: World Bank Institute, 1999), and *Les*

Solutions emergentes (Emerging Solutions) (Quebec: Clair Commission of Study for Health and Social Services Report, January 2001).

73 Cited by Matthew Miller, "A Bold Experiment to Fix City Schools," *Atlantic Monthly* 284, 1 (July 1999), Part 2, pp. 15–18 and pp. 26–31, 27.

74 It is interesting — and revealing — that vouchers and charters have figured so prominently in the current debate about public education. There are, after all, several possible ways of creating public markets in education. Governments, acting on behalf of citizens, could finance private — either for-profit or not-for-profit — suppliers, who would compete for government contracts to provide public education. This is largely the story of public markets in health care, and it is also how schools in Canada, New Zealand, Australia, and the United Kingdom were financed in the early nineteenth century. This kind of plan, however, would not give parents choice.

75 Girard, "Schoolhouse Dues."

76 Jeffrey Henig, *Rethinking School Choice: Limits of the Market Metaphor* (Princeton, NJ: Princeton University Press, 1994).

77 Jodi Wilgoren, "Schools Are Now Marketers Where Choice Is Taking Hold," *New York Times*, April 20, 2001, pp. A1, A12.

78 Gratzer, *Code Blue*, p. 182.

Chapter IV: Measuring Up: Constructing Accountability

1 Interview of David Naylor, *Medicare in Crisis*, p. 4.

2 Cited in Schofield et al., "Saving Our Schools."

3 Margaret Wente, "Everyone Is Nicely Off Hook in Death

of Baby," *Globe and Mail*, April 12, 2001, pp. A1, A20.

4 David Held, *Models of Democracy*, 2d ed. (Stanford, CA: Stanford University Press, 1996), p. 27.

5 Xenophon, *History of Greece*, 1.7, in C. Rodewald, ed., *Democracy: Ideas and Realities* (London: Dent, 1974), pp. 1–6, 2.

6 Michael J. Trebilcock, *The Prospects for Reinventing Government* (Toronto: C. D. Howe Institute, 1994), p. 8.

7 Max Weber, "Politics As a Vocation," in H. H. Gerth and C. W. Mills, eds., *From Max Weber* (New York: Oxford University Press, 1972), pp. 77–128, 113.

8 Held, *Models of Democracy*, pp. 172–73.

9 C. B. Macpherson, *The Real World of Democracy* (Toronto: CBC, 1965; Anansi, 1992), and Carole Pateman, *Participation and Democratic Theory* (Cambridge: Cambridge University Press, 1970).

10 For a discussion of the state as "steering" rather than "rowing," see David Osborne and Ted Gaebler, *Reinventing Government* (New York: Plume, 1993).

11 Colleen Flood, *International Health Care Reform: A Legal, Economic, and Political Analysis* (London: New York, 2000), p. 130, and *Accountability of Health Service Purchasers* (Toronto: Centre for the Study of State and Market, University of Toronto, 1997), p. 3.

12 J. D. Donahue, *The Privatization Decision: Public Ends, Private Means* (New York: Basic Books, 1989), p. 10.

13 This need not be the case: in Alberta, charter school students are tested in the same way as students in the regular public system.

14 Alan Maynard, "Competition and Quality: Rhetoric and Reality," *International Journal for Quality in Health Care* 10, 5 (1998), pp. 379–84.

15 Flood, *Accountability of Health Service Purchasers*, p. 16.

16 Terry Moe at a seminar in Sacramento in 1999, cited by Bruce Fuller, *Inside Charter Schools: The Paradox of Radical Decentralization* (Cambridge, MA: Harvard University Press, 2000), p. 238.

17 Economists and rational-choice theorists, who measure utility subjectively, give great weight to satisfaction.

18 On "the vital issue of accountability," says Radwanski, "there can be no effective pursuit of excellence in educational outcomes without meaningful accountability, and there can be no meaningful accountability without measurable standards of accomplishment." George Radwanski, *Ontario Study of the Relevance of Education and the Issue of Dropouts* (Toronto: Ministry of Education, 1987), p. 56, cited in Ronald Manzer, *Public Schools and Political Ideas: Canadian Educational Policy in Historical Perspective* (Toronto: University of Toronto Press, 1994), p. 227.

19 The Third International Mathematics and Science Study (TIMSS) was done in the 1990s. Harold Stevenson, "A TIMSS Primer," *Fordham Report*, 2, 7 (1998), pp. 1–28.

20 The Council of Ministers for Education in Canada, created by the provinces, introduced the School Achievement Indicators Project in 1989. Manzer, *Public Schools and Political Ideas*, p. 245. For an excellent review of the multiple difficulties of using test results as a measure of school effectiveness, see Sajitha Basir, "The Cost-Effectiveness of Public and Private Schools: Knowledge Gaps, New Research Methodologies, and an Application in India," in Christopher Colclough, ed., *Marketizing Education and Health in Developing Countries* (Oxford: Clarendon Press, 1997), pp. 124–64.

21 Alberta, British Columbia, and New Brunswick release

annual data on school performance based on standardized testing. Ontario has introduced a new compulsory
curriculum, new report cards, mandatory testing of the literacy and numeracy of students in primary and
secondary school, and mandatory testing of teachers.

22 Norman Frederiksen, a specialist with the Educational
Testing Service, cited by Alfie Kohn, *The Schools Our Children Deserve* (Boston: Houghton Mifflin, 1999), p. 75.

23 Mumford, *Pentagon of Power*, vol. 2, p. 184.

24 Jodi Wilgoren, "Possible Cheating Scandal Is Investigated
in Michigan," *New York Times*, June 9, 2001, p. A7. A seemingly trivial but related problem is human error in scoring
the tests. Even though the tests are simple to score, error
has plagued the testing industry in the past several years
as demand for its services have grown and its capacity has
been stretched. One programming error led to 9,000 students in New York City being mistakenly forced to go to
summer school and the firing of five of thirty-two neighbourhood school superintendents by Dr. Rudy Crew, the
chancellor of education in New York State. He himself lost
his job over falling scores before the error was discovered.
Human error is inevitable, but small errors have large consequences as they ripple through the lives of schools and
students. Jacques Steinberg and Diana Henriques, "When
a Test Fails the Schools, Careers and Reputations Suffer,"
New York Times, May 21, 2001, pp. A1, A10–11, and
Henriques and Steinberg, "Right Answer, Wrong Score:
Test Flaws Take Toll," *New York Times*, May 20, 2001, pp.
A1, A22–23. This is a cautionary tale of the dangers of rely-
ing on a small group of private companies to hold those
who deliver public goods accountable.

25 Stevenson, "A TIMMS Primer," p. 1.

26 Richard Atkinson, "Excerpt from a Speech to the Annual Meeting of the Council on Higher Education on New S.A.T. Policy," *New York Times*, Feb. 17, 2001, p. A13.

27 Jo Ann Boyston, ed., *The Collected Works of John Dewey: Later Works*, vol. II (Carbondale: Southern Illinois University Press, 1987), p. 240.

28 John Ralston Saul, *The Unconscious Civilization* (Toronto: Anansi, 1995), p. 65.

29 "Traditional standardized testing in education," argues Monty Neil, the executive director of the National Center for Fair and Open Testing, "has had predominantly harmful social consequences." The damage is most severe to students from low-income families and minority groups. "The often incorrect presumptions are then made," Neil continues, "that these students cannot learn well and that they need a stronger dose of what demonstrably has not worked." Neill, *How the Principles and Indicators for Student Assessment Systems Should Affect Practice* (Cambridge, MA: National Center for Fair and Open Testing, 1996), p. 3. Available at fairtest.org.

30 Cited in Schofield, "Saving Our Schools," and Michael Fullan, *The New Meaning of Educational Change*, 3rd ed. (New York: Teachers College Press, 2001).

31 Interview with Michael Fullan, Toronto, April 10, 2001. The British government has targeted funding to those schools that need it most, and reinforced new resources with intensive professional development for teachers. The strategy seems to be working: the percentage of eleven-year-olds scoring in the top two levels of the national literacy test rose from 56 percent in 1996 to 75 percent in 2000. Schofield, "Saving Our Schools." In Texas, the focus on more clearly articulated standards, tighter tracking of

low-performing schools, and early intervention in reading helped close the gap between white, Latino, and African-American students. Fuller, *Inside Charter Schools*, p. 57.

32 Fullan, *New Meaning of Educational Change*, pp. 220-24.

33 Tests of this kind are "norm-referenced": they measure how a student is performing in comparison with others. "Criterion-referenced" tests measure students against a yardstick, rather than against one another.

34 Peter Cowley and Shahrokh Shahabi-Azad, *The Report Card on Ontario's Secondary Schools* (Vancouver: Fraser Institute, 2001).

35 Louise Brown, "Demographics Play Role in Literacy Scores," *Toronto Star*, April 10, 2001, p. B4.

36 Louise Brown, "Grading System Targets Neediest Schools," *Toronto Star*, June 10, 2001, pp. A1, A6.

37 The four states with large numbers of charter schools — Florida, Minnesota, North Carolina, and Wisconsin — recently reported less than 55 percent monitoring of student achievement. Berman et al., *The State of Charter Schools 2000*, p. 50.

38 Chester Finn et al., *Charter Schools in Action: Final Report*, Part 4 (New York: The Hudson Institute, 1997), pp. 1–2. Available at www.edexcellence.net/chart/chart4.htm.

39 In wealthy Marin County in California, where students have done very well on the tests in the past, nearly 20 percent got parental waivers releasing them from taking the state tests. As a result, the school district will be ineligible for state bonuses. The same kind of revolt is growing in Scarsdale and Rochester, in New York, among more affluent parents. Richard Rothstein, "The Growing Revolt Against the Testers," *New York Times*, May 30, 2001, p. A19.

40 Wente, "Everyone is Nicely Off Hook in Death of Baby."

41 Richard G. Wilkinson, *Unhealthy Societies: The Afflictions of Inequality* (London: Routledge, 1996).

42 Personal e-mail to the author, June 5, 2001.

43 Interview of Terry Sullivan, "Time for Health Guides and Report Cards?" *The Atkinson Letter* (Toronto: The Atkinson Foundation, Winter 1999), p. 2.

44 A. L. Cochrane, *Effectiveness and Efficiency: Random Reflections on Health Services* (London: Nuffield Provincial Hospitals Trust, 1972).

45 J. Green, N. Wintfeld, P. Sharkey, and L. J. Passman, "The Importance of Severity of Illness in Assessing Hospital Mortality," *Journal of the American Medical Association* 263, 2 (1990), pp. 241–46. The sophisticated and successful adjustments for case mix that do exist — such as APACHE II, used in intensive care — are rare exceptions.

46 J. Mant and N. Hicks, "Detecting Differences in the Quality of Care: the Sensitivity of Measures of Process and Outcome in Treating Acute Myocardial Infarction," *British Medical Journal* 311, 7008 (1995), pp. 793–97. In most kinds of health care delivered in hospitals, outcomes have to be assessed with measures such as the status of the disease, functional ability, and quality of life. These measures, especially the last, are often difficult to assess with precision. Generally, there are only weak statistical associations between care processes and outcomes.

47 André Picard, "Health Centre to Push Doctors to Make Use of Best Research," *Globe and Mail*, July 3, 2001, p. A8.

48 Interview with author, Toronto, February 18, 2001.

49 Susan Rappolt, "Clinical Guidelines and the Fate of Medical Autonomy in Ontario," *Social Science and Medicine* 44, 7 (1997), pp. 977–87, and Tuohy, *Accidental Logics*, pp. 220–22.

50 Cited by Picard, "Health Centre to Push Doctors."

51 Cost-cutting in the acute-care sector over the past decade was in part deliberate. Analysts of the Canadian health-care system warned again and again that too many resources were being invested in the hospital sector — where costs per patient are very high — and too few in other institutions that could provide supportive but much less expensive care. The best available evidence shows that some hospitals have become more cost-effective: they treat as many, and in some cases more, patients than they did before beds were closed; the average length of stay in hospital has gone down 24 percent in the past decade; and death rates after surgery did not increase. The Atkinson Letter, "Interview with Noralou Roos," *Medicare in Crisis: Myths and Realities*, vol. 2 (Toronto: Atkinson Foundation, 1996), p. 1, and *Medicare in Crisis* (Jan. 10, 1997), p. 3.

52 In the past decade, as health-care costs continued to rise, governments tried to improve the efficiency of hospitals. Real per capita spending on hospitals in Canada did decrease by 7.2 percent from 1990 to 1996, while total real per capita health spending increased by 1.7 percent during the same period. The hospital share of total health expenditures decreased from 38.2 percent in 1990 to 34.9 percent in 1996. This drop of 3.3 percent over six years compares to a drop of 7 percent over the preceding twenty years. Tuohy, *Accidental Logics*, p. 213.

53 More generically, all systems, when faced with the imperative to contain spending, have strong tendencies to shift costs rather than to improve performance. Accountability becomes especially important under these conditions. Colleen Flood, "Accountability, Flexibility, and Integration," *Policy Options* 21, 4 (May 2000), pp. 17–19.

54 The report cards are done by the University of Toronto
    and published by the Canadian Institute for Health Infor-
    mation, a national, not-for-profit health-information
    organization. *Hospital Report 98*, *Hospital Report 99*, and
    Hospital Report 2001 examine performance in four major
    sectors of hospital activity: patient satisfaction, patient
    care, hospital finances, and system integration and
    change. See www.utoronto.ca/hlthadmn.

55 Interview of Terry Sullivan, "Time for Health Guides and
    Report Cards?"

56 Waiting times are private costs, and they are not included
    in any cost analysis. Canadian Institute for Health Infor-
    mation, *Health Care in Canada* (Ottawa: Statistics Canada,
    2001), p. 31, and Carolyn Tuohy, Colleen Flood, and Mark
    Stabile, *How Does Private Finance Affect Public Health Care
    Systems?* (University of Toronto working paper, March
    2001), pp. 11–13.

57 Interview of Terry Sullivan, *The Atkinson Letter, Health Care
    Reform: Lost Opportunity — Part 1* (Toronto: The Atkinson
    Foundation, Oct. 2000), p. 2.

58 Marko Simunovic, Anna Gagliardi, David McCready,
    Angela Coates, Mark Levine, and Denny DePetrillo, "A
    Snapshot of Waiting Times for Cancer Surgery Provided
    by Surgeons Affiliated with Cancer Centres in Ontario,"
    Canadian Medical Association Journal 165, 4 (Aug. 21, 2001),
    pp. 421–25.

59 Interview of Lisa Priest, "Time for Health Guides and
    Report Cards?" *The Atkinson Letter* (Winter 1999), p. 2.

60 Lisa Priest, *Operating in the Dark: Accountability in Our
    Health Care System* (Toronto: The Atkinson Foundation,
    1999), p. 4.

61 Public accountability has also contributed to a significant

improvement in outcomes: risk-adjusted death for coronary artery bypass graft surgery dropped significantly after report cards were issued regularly.

62 Every province does hospital-by-hospital analyses of major procedures. There is no shortage of good evidence, but the evidence is very technical and reports are not written for the general public. The Institute for Clinical Evaluation Sciences (ICES) in Ontario has released a report card on survival rates at hospitals for cardiac patients. It continues to do work on hospital practices, variation of services by region, and patterns of use. Interview of Terry Sullivan, "Time for Health Guides and Report Cards?"

63 Provincial colleges of physicians and surgeons rely largely on information that the doctors themselves provide. Ninety-nine percent of the 13,000 complaints investigated by the College of Physicians and Surgeons in Ontario in the past six years were either dismissed or handled in secrecy. An investigation into the college's system of accountability found a system "that typically hands out lenient penalties, rarely revokes licenses, can take years to render decisions, and puts doctors on higher legal footing than complainants." Robert Cribb, Rita Daly, and Laurie Monsebraaten, "How System Helps Shield Bad Doctors," *Toronto Star*, May 5, 2001, pp. A1, A14, and Rita Daly, Robert Cribb, and Laurie Monsebraaten, "MDs Face New Bid to End Secrecy," *Toronto Star*, May 7, 2001, pp. A1, A6–7.

64 Laurie Monsebraaten, Rita Daly, and Robert Cribb, "Ontario Examines Doctor Secrecy," *Toronto Star*, May 6, 2001, pp. A1, A6–7.

65 Gay Abbate, "MDs Need Oversight From Public, Report

Says," *Globe and Mail*, June 25, 2001, pp. A1, A7.

66   Cited by Laurie Monsebraaten, Rita Daly, and Robert Cribb, "Ontario Examines Doctor Secrecy."

67   The College of Physicians and Surgeons in Ontario, a self-regulating body, conducts random assessments of a small number of physicians annually in an effort to catch problem doctors before they harm patients. The annual assessments cover no more than 550 of 20,000 practising physicians. At this rate, a doctor could practise for forty years before being assessed.

68   In Massachusetts, the public reporting of physician performance was negotiated with the physicians' association. Since the association was at the table — and actually sponsored the legislation — doctors have complained very little about the new level of reporting to the public.

69   M. A. Thomson O'Brien, A. D. Oxman, R. B. Haynes, D. A. Davis, N. Freemantle, and E. L. Harvey, "Local Opinion Leaders: Effects on Professional Practice and Health Care Outcomes," *Cochrane Review 2001*, Cochrane Database System Rev. CD000125.

70   Personal e-mail to the author, June 5, 2001.

Chapter V: The Culture of Choice

1   G. K. Chesterton, *Orthodoxy* (New York: Dodd, Mead, 1908; republished New York: Image Books, Doubleday, 1990), p. 81. My thanks to Philip Siller for this citation.

2   Heath, *Efficient Society*, p. 300.

3   The first Social Accountability Code (SA 8000) was introduced by non-governmental organizations in 1998, on the fiftieth anniversary of the Universal Declaration of Human Rights.

4   Danilo Zolo, *Democracy and Complexity*, David McKie, trans. (Cambridge: Polity Press, 1992), p. 54.

5   Philip Allott, "Behind Voter Apathy, A Silent Revolution," *International Herald Tribune*, June 6, 2001.

6   Chesterton, *Orthodoxy*, p. 81.

7   Cited by Robert B. Reich, "The Choice Fetish," *Civilization* 7, 4 (Aug. 2000), pp. 64–66.

8   Heath, *Efficient Society*, pp. viii, 7.

9   Negri and Michael Hardt, *Empire*, pp. 280–82.

10 Ibid.

11 Alan Wolfe, "The Final Freedom," *New York Times Magazine*, Mar. 18, 2001, pp. 48–51.

12 F. A. Hayek, *The Constitution of Liberty* (London: Routledge and Kegan Paul, 1960), p. 12.

13 Claudia Mills, "Choice and Circumstance," *Ethics* 109, 1 (Oct. 1998), pp. 154–65.

14 John Stuart Mill, *On Liberty* (London: Oxford University Press, 1972), p. 15.

15 Andrew Reeve, "Individual Choice and the Retreat from Utilitarianism," in Lincoln Allison, ed., *The Utilitarian Response: The Contemporary Viability of Utilitarian Political Philosophy* (London: Jay, 1990), pp. 98–119, 103.

16 Deborah Stone, in *Policy Paradox and Political Reason*, pp. 87–103, frames the question this way.

17 Jack Donnelly, *The Concept of Human Rights* (London: Croom Helm, 1985), and *Universal Human Rights in Theory and Practice* (Ithaca, NY: Cornell University Press, 1989).

18 Here, negative substantive rights are very similar to Isaiah Berlin's concept of negative liberty. See "Two Concepts of Liberty," in his *Four Essays on Liberty* (New York: Oxford University Press, 1969), pp. 118–72.

19 Ronald Green, "Health Care and Justice in Contract

Theory Perspective," in Robert Veatch and Roy Branson, eds., *Ethics and Health Policy* (Cambridge, MA: Ballinger, 1976), pp. 111–26.

20 Roy Bhaskar, *The Possibility of Naturalism* (New Brunswick, NJ: Humanities Press, 1979), p. 43.

21 Ignatieff, *The Rights Revolution*, p. 2.

22 Macpherson, *The Real World of Democracy*.

23 I am indebted to Melissa Williams for the distinction between the right to choice as commitment and as possibility.

24 Robert Nozick, *Anarchy, State, and Utopia* (New York: Basic Books, 1974). The procedural conditions set limits on processes of acquisition and transfer.

25 John Rawls, *A Theory of Justice* (Cambridge: Harvard University Press, 1971).

26 Ibid, p. 62. Moreover, social and economic inequalities attached to offices and positions must be open to all.

27 Ibid, pp. 266–70.

28 Stone, *Policy Paradox and Political Reason*, p. 136.

29 Economists would describe this kind of process as revealing preferences. Society as a whole, argues Joseph Raz, provides choices so that individuals can discover themselves. *The Morality of Freedom* (Oxford: Clarendon Press, 1986).

30 Antonio R. Damasio, *Descartes' Error: Emotion, Reason, and the Human Brain* (New York: Putnam, 1994).

31 Mills, "Choice and Circumstance," pp. 154–65, 154, 157.

32 Ibid, p. 163.

33 Hirschman, *Exit, Voice, and Loyalty*.

34 Heath, *Efficient Society*, pp. 58–59.

35 Reich, "The Choice Fetish," p. 66.

36 Jürgen Habermas, *Between Facts and Norms: Contributions*

to a Discourse Theory of Law and Democracy, William Rehg,
trans. (Cambridge, MA: MIT Press, 1996).

Postscript: Security in the Post-industrial Age

1 Charles Tilly, "Reflections on the History of European State-Making." In Charles Tilly, ed., *The Formation of National States in Western Europe* (Princeton, NJ: Princeton University Press, 1975), pp. 3–83.

2 Arthur Schlesinger, *The Imperial Presidency* (Boston: Houghton Mifflin, 1973).

3 Manuel Castells, *The Rise of the Network Society*, vol. 1 of *The Information Age: Economy, Society, and Culture* (Oxford: Blackwell, 1996), p. 469.

4 Janice Gross Stein, Richard Stren, Joy Fitzgibbon, and Melissa MacLean, *Networks of Knowledge: Collaborative Innovations in International Learning* (Toronto: University of Toronto Press, 2001).

5 Cited in David J. Garrow, "Another Lesson From World War II Internments," *New York Times*, September 23, 2001, 4, p. 6.

BIBLIOGRAPHY

Abramson, Paul, and Ronald Inglehart. *Value Change in Global Perspective*. Ann Arbor: University of Michigan Press, 1995.

Allen, William H. *Efficient Democracy*. New York: Dodd, Mead and Co., 1907.

Alvin, M., and M. Sverke. "Do New Generations Imply the End of Solidarity? Swedish Unionism in the Era of Individualization." *Economic and Industrial Democracy* 21, 1 (2000): 71–95.

Arthurs, H. W. "Globalization of the Mind: Canadian Elites and the Restructuring of Legal Fields." *Canadian Journal of Law and Society* 12, 2 (1997): 219–46.

The Atkinson Letter, *Health Care Reform: Lost Opportunity — Part 1*. Toronto: The Atkinson Foundation, 2000.

——. *Medicare in Crisis: Myths and Realities*. Toronto: The Atkinson Foundation, 1996, 1997.

——. *Time for Health Guides and Report Cards?* Toronto: The Atkinson Foundation, 1999.

Banting, Keith. "The Internationalization of the Social Contract." In *The Nation-state in a Global/Information Era: Policy Challenges*, edited by Thomas Courchene.

Kingston: John Deutsch Institute for Economic Research, 1999.

Barnes, Samuel, Max Kaase, Klaus Allerbeck, Barbara G. Farah, Felix Heunks, Ronald Inglehart, M. Kent Jennings, Hans D. Klingemann, Allan Marsh, and Leopold Rosenmayr. *Political Action: Mass Participation in Five Western Democracies*. Beverly Hills: Sage Publications, 1979.

Barzelay, Michael. *Breaking through Bureaucracy: A New Vision for Managing in Government*. Berkeley: University of California Press, 1992.

Basir, Sajitha. "The Cost-Effectiveness of Public and Private Schools: Knowledge Gaps, New Research Methodologies, and an Application in India." In *Marketizing Education and Health in Developing Countries*, edited by Christopher Colclough. Oxford: Clarendon Press, 1997.

Bell, Daniel. *The Coming of Post-industrial Society*. New York: Basic Books, 1973.

———. *The Cultural Contradictions of Capitalism*. New York: Basic Books, 1976.

Bentham, Jeremy. *Economic Writings*. 3 vols. Edited by W. Stark. London: Allen and Unwin, 1952–54.

———. *A Fragment on Government and an Introduction to Principles of Morals and Legislation*. Edited by Wilfred Harrison. Oxford: Blackwell, 1967.

———. *Principles of Morals and Legislation*. Edited by J. H. Burns and H. L. A. Hart. Oxford: Clarendon Press, 1996.

Berlin, Isaiah. "Two Concepts of Liberty." In *Four Essays on Liberty*. New York: Oxford University Press, 1969.

Berman, Paul, et al. *The State of Charter Schools 2000: Fourth-Year Report*. Washington, D.C.: U.S. Department of Education, Office of Educational Research and Development, 2000.

Bhaskar, Roy. *The Possibility of Naturalism*. New Brunswick, NJ: Humanities Press, 1979.

Bishop, John H. "Privatizing Education: Lessons from Canada and Europe." In *Vouchers and the Provision of Public Services*, edited by C. Eugene Steuerle, Van Doorn Ooms, George Peterson, and Robert D. Reischauer. Washington, D.C.: Brookings Institution, 2000.

Blanchard, Lloyd A., Charles C. Hinnant, and Wilson Wong. "Market-Based Reforms: Toward a Social Subcontract?" *Administration and Society* 30, 5 (1998): 483–512.

Blendon, Robert, Karen Donelan, Cathy Schoen, Karen Davis, and Katherine Binns. "The Cost of Health System Change: Public Discontent in Five Nations." *Health Affairs* 18, 3 (May/June 1999): 206–16.

Bosetti, Lynn. "Alberta Charter Schools: Paradox and Promises." *Alberta Journal of Educational Research* 66, 2 (Summer 2000): 179–90.

——. "The Dark Promise of Charter Schools." *Policy Options* 19, 6 (July–Aug. 1998): 63–67.

Bosetti, Lynn, et al. *Canadian Charter Schools at the Crossroads: Executive Summary*. Kelowna, BC: Society for the Advancement of Excellence in Education, 2000.

Bosworth, David. "The Spirit of Capitalism 2000." *The Public Interest* 138 (Winter, 2000): 3–28.

Boyston, Jo Ann, ed. *The Collected Works of John Dewey: Later Works Volume 1–18*. Carbondale: Southern Illinois University Press, 1987.

Buchanan, James M., and Robert D. Tollison, eds. *Theory of Public Choice: Political Application of Economics*. Ann Arbor: University of Michigan Press, 1972.

Buechler, M. *Charter Schools: Legislation and Results After Four Years*. Bloomington: Indiana Education Policy Center, 1995.

Canadian Institute for Health Information. *Health Care in Canada*. Ottawa: Statistics Canada, 2001.

Carson, Rachel. *Silent Spring*. Greenwich, CT: Fawcett, 1962.

Caesar, James W., and Patrick J. McGuinn. "Civic Education Reconsidered." *The Public Interest* 133 (Fall 1998): 84–103.

Castells, Manuel. *The Rise of the Network Society*. Oxford: Blackwell, 1990.

Cerny, Philip. "Globalization and Other Stories: The Search for a New Paradigm for International Relations." *International Journal* 51, 4 (1996): 617–37.

Chesterton, G. K. *Orthodoxy*. New York: Dodd, Mead, 1908. Reprint. New York: Image Books, Doubleday, 1990.

Chubb, John, and Terry Moe. *Politics, Markets, and America's Schools*. Washington, D.C.: Brookings Institution, 1990.

Clair Commission. *Les Solutions emergentes* (Emerging Solutions). Quebec: Clair Commission of Study for Health and Social Services, 2001.

Cochrane, A. L. *Effectiveness and Efficiency: Random Reflections on Health Services*. London: Nuffield Provincial Hospitals Trust, 1972.

Coleman, James S., Ernest R. Campbell, Carol S. Hobson, James McPartland, Alexander M. Mood, Frederic D. Weinfeld, and Robert L. York. *Equality of Educational Opportunity*. Washington, D.C.: Department of Health, Education, and Welfare, 1966.

Coleman, William. "The Project on Trends: An Introduction." *Canadian Public Policy* 26 (2000): 1–14.

Courchene, Thomas, and John N. McDougall. "The Context for Future Constitutional Options." In *Options for a New Canada*, edited by Ronald B. Watts and Douglas M. Brown. Toronto: University of Toronto Press, 1991.

Cowley, Peter and Shahrokh Shahabi-Azad. *Report Card*

on Ontario's Secondary Schools. Vancouver: Fraser Institute, 2001.

Damasio, Antonio R. *Descartes' Error: Emotion, Reason, and the Human Brain*. New York: Putnam, 1994.

Deber, Raisa. "Getting What We Pay For: Myths and Realities about Financing Canada's Health Care System." Paper prepared for the National Dialogue on Health Reform, April 11, 2000.

———. "Medical Savings Accounts: A Fine Idea Unless You're Sick." *Health Policy Forum* (Spring 1999): 4–5.

DeCoster, Carolyn, K. C. Carriere, Sandra Peterson, Randy Wald, and Leonard MacWilliam. *Surgical Waiting Times in Manitoba*. Winnipeg: Manitoba Centre for Health Policy and Evaluation, 1998.

Dicksee, Lawrence R. *The True Basis of Efficiency*. London: Gee, 1922.

Donahue, J. D. *The Privatization Decision: Public Ends, Private Means*. New York: Basic Books, 1989.

Donaldson, Cam, Gillian Currie, and Craig Milton. *Integrating Canada's Dis-Integrated Health Care System*. Toronto: C. D. Howe Institute, 2001.

Donnelly, Jack. *The Concept of Human Rights*. London: Croom Helm, 1985.

———. *Universal Human Rights in Theory and Practice*. Ithaca, NY: Cornell University Press, 1989.

Downs, Anthony. *An Economic Theory of Democracy*. New York: Harper and Row, 1957.

Economic Council of Canada. *A Lot to Learn: Education and Training in Canada*. Ottawa: Minister of Supply and Services Canada, 1992.

Ester, Peter, Leok Halman, and Ruud de Moor. "Value Shift in Western Societies." In *The Individualizing Society: Value Change in Europe and North America*, edited by Ester, Halman and de Moor. Tilburg, Neth.: Tilburg University Press, 1993.

Feldberg, Gina and Robert Vipond. "The Virus of Con-
    sumerism." In *Market Limits in Health Reform: Public
    Success, Private Failure*, edited by Daniel Drache
    and Terry Sullivan. London: Routledge, 1999.

Ferguson, Yale, and Richard Mansbach. *Polities: Authority,
    Identities, and Change*. Columbia, SC: University of
    South Carolina Press, 1996.

Finn, Chester E., Jr., Bruno V. Manno, and Gregg
    Vanourek. *Charter Schools in Action: Renewing Public
    Education*. Princeton, NJ: Princeton University Press,
    2000.

——. *Charter Schools in Action: Final Report, Part* 4.
    New York: The Hudson Institute, 1997.

Flood, Colleen. "Accountability, Flexibility, and Integra-
    tion." *Policy Options* 21, 4 (May 2000): 17–19.

——. *Accountability of Health Service Purchasers*. Toronto:
    Centre for the Study of State and Market, University of
    Toronto, 1997.

——. *International Health Care Reform: A Legal, Economic,
    and Political Analysis*. London: Routledge, 1999.

Friedman, Milton. "The Role of Government in Educa-
    tion." In *Economics and the Public Interest*, edited by
    Robert A. Solow. New Brunswick, NJ: Rutgers Press,
    1955.

Fukuyama, Francis. *The End of History and the Last Man*.
    New York: Avon, 1992.

——. *Trust: The Social Virtues and the Creation of Prosperity*.
    New York: The Free Press, 1995.

Fullan, Michael. *The New Meaning of Educational Change*.
    New York: Teachers College Press, 2001.

Fuller, Bruce J. *Inside Charter Schools: The Paradox of Radical
    Decentralization*. Cambridge, MA: Harvard University
    Press, 2000.

Gardner, J. "Medical Savings Accounts Make Waves."
    Modern Healthcare 25, 9 (1995): 57–62.

Garrett, Geoffrey. "Global Markets and National Politics: Collision Course or Virtuous Circle." *International Organization* 52, 4 (1998): 787–824.

Garrett, Geoffrey, and Peter Lange. "Internationalization, Institutions, and Political Change." In *Internationalization and Domestic Politics*, edited by Helen Milner and Robert Keohane. Cambridge: Cambridge University Press, 1996.

Gratzer, David. *Code Blue: Reviving Canada's Health Care System*. Toronto: ECW Press, 1999.

Gray, John. *Hayek on Liberty*. Oxford: Blackwell, 1984.

Green, J., N. Wintfeld, P. Sharkey, and L. J. Passman. "The Importance of Severity of Illness in Assessing Hospital Mortality." *Journal of the American Medical Association* 263, 2 (1990): 241–46

Green, Ronald. "Health Care and Justice in Contract Theory Perspective." In *Ethics and Health Policy*, edited by Robert Veatch and Roy Branson. Cambridge, MA: Ballinger, 1976.

Greene, Jay, Paul Peterson, and J. Du. "Effectiveness of School Choice: The Milwaukee Experiment." Department of Government, Harvard University, 1997. Unpublished report.

Gregg, Allan R. "A Shifting Landscape." *Maclean's* 113/114, 52/1 (Dec. 25, 2000/Jan.1, 2001): 31–35.

Greven, Michael Th. and Louis W. Pauly, eds. *Democracy Beyond the State? The European Dilemma and the Emerging Global Order*. Latham, MD: Rowman and Littlefield, 2000.

Habermas, Jürgen. *Between Facts and Norms: Contributions to a Discourse Theory of Law and Democracy*, translated by William Rehg. Cambridge, MA: MIT Press, 1996.

Hanushek, Eric. "The Economics of Schooling: Production and Efficiency in Public Schools." *Journal of Economic Literature* 24, 3 (Sept. 1986): 1141–77.

Hayek, F. A. *The Constitution of Liberty*. London: Routledge and Kegan Paul, 1960.

Heath, Joseph. *The Efficient Society: Why Canada Is as Close to Utopia as It Gets*. Toronto: Penguin, 2001.

Held, David. *Democracy and the Global Order: From the Modern State to Cosmopolitan Governance*. Stanford, CA: Stanford University Press, 1995.

——. *Global Transformations*. Stanford, CA: Stanford University Press, 1999.

——. *Models of Democracy*. 2d ed. Stanford, CA: Stanford University Press, 1996.

Helliwell, John. *Globalization: Myths, Facts, and Consequences*. Toronto: C. D. Howe Institute, 2000.

Henig, Jeffrey. *Rethinking School Choice: Limits of the Market Metaphor*. Princeton, NJ: Princeton University Press, 1994.

Hepburn, Claudia R., ed. *Can the Markets Save Our Schools?* Vancouver: Fraser Institute, 2001.

Hirschman, Albert O. *Exit, Voice, and Loyalty: Responses to Decline in Firms, Organizations, and States*. Cambridge, MA: Harvard University Press, 1970.

——. *Rival Views of Market Society and Other Recent Essays*. New York: Viking, 1986.

Holmes, Stephen. "The Secret History of Self-Interest." In *Beyond Self-Interest*, edited by Jane J. Mansbridge. Chicago: University of Chicago Press, 1990.

Hsiao, W. "Medical Savings Accounts: Lessons from Singapore." *Health Affairs* 14, 2 (1995): 260–66.

Hurrell, A., and N. Woods. "Globalization and Inequality." *Millennium* 24, 3 (1995): 447–70.

Ignatieff, Michael. *The Rights Revolution*. Toronto: Anansi, 2000.

Inglehart, Ronald. *Modernization and Postmodernization: Cultural, Economic, and Political Change in 43 Societies*. Princeton, NJ: Princeton University Press, 1997.

Institute for Research on Public Policy (IRPP). *IRPP Task Force on Health Policy: Recommendations to First Ministers*. Montreal: IRPP, 2000.

Investing in Students Task Force. *Portals and Pathways: A Review of Post-Secondary Education in Ontario*. Toronto: Queen's Park, 2001.

Izu, Joanne, et al. *Cross-Site Report: An Evaluation of Charter Schools in Los Angeles Unified School District*. San Francisco: WestEd, 1998.

Jérôme-Forget, Monique, Joseph White, and Joshua M. Wiener, eds. *Health Care Reform through Internal Markets: Experience and Proposals*. Montreal: IRPP, 1995.

Kahne, Joseph. "Democratic Communities, Equity, and Excellence: A Deweyan Reframing of Educational Policy Analysis." *Educational Evaluation and Policy Analysis* 3, 16 (Fall 1994): 233–48.

Klein, R., and J. Dixon. "Cash Bonanza for NHS: The Price Is Centralization." *British Medical Journal* 320, 7239 (2000): 883–84.

Kohn, Alfie. *The Schools Our Children Deserve*. Boston: Houghton Mifflin, 1999.

Lebow, Richard Ned, and Janice Gross Stein. *We All Lost the Cold War*. Princeton, NJ: Princeton University Press, 1991.

Leonard, Mark. "The Left Should Love Globalization." *New Statesman* (May 28, 2001): 36–37.

Lowi, Theodore, and Edward J. Harpham. "Political Theory and Public Policy." In *Contemporary Empirical Political Theory*, edited by Kristen R. Monroe. Berkeley: University of California Press, 1997.

Lowry, S. Todd. *The Archaeology of Economic Ideas: The Classical Greek Tradition*. Durham, NC: Duke University Press, 1987.

Macpherson, C. B. *The Real World of Democracy*. Toronto: CBC, 1965; Anansi, 1992.

Mant, J., and N. Hicks. "Detecting Differences in the Quality of Care: The Sensitivity of Measures of Process and Outcome in Treating Acute Myocardial Infarction." *British Medical Journal* 311, 7008 (1995): 793–97.

Manzer, Ronald. *Public Schools and Political Ideas: Canadian Educational Policy in Historical Perspective.* Toronto: University of Toronto Press, 1994.

Marshall, Robert. "Paying the Price." *Maclean's* 113/114, 1/52 (Dec. 25, 2000/Jan. 1, 2001): 48–50.

Massero, T. A., and Y. Wong. "Positive Experience with Medical Savings Accounts in Singapore." *Health Affairs* 14, 2 (1995): 267–72.

Matthews, David. "Public Government/Public Schools." *National Civic Review* 85, 3 (Fall 1996): 14–22.

Maynard, Alan. "Competition and Quality: Rhetoric and Reality." *International Journal for Quality in Health Care* 10, 5 (1998): 379–84.

McArthur, William, Cynthia Ramsay, and Michael Walker, eds. *Healthy Incentives: Canadian Health Reform in an International Context.* Vancouver: Fraser Institute, 1996.

McMahon, Fred. "Public Funding with Market Dynamics." *Policy Options* 21, 4 (May 2000): 9–11.

Meek, Roland L., and Andres S. Skinner. "The Development of Adam Smith's Ideas on the Division of Labour." *Economic Journal* 88, 332 (1973): 1094–116.

Mill, John Stuart. *On Liberty.* London: Oxford University Press, 1972.

Miller, Matthew. "A Bold Experiment to Fix City Schools." Part 2. *Atlantic Monthly* 284, 1 (July 1999): 15–18, 26–31.

Mills, Claudia. "Choice and Circumstance." *Ethics* 109, 1 (Oct. 1998): 154–65.

Monroe, Kristen R. "Human Nature, Identity, and Politics." In *Contemporary Empirical Political Theory,* edited by Kristen R. Monroe. Berkeley: University of California Press, 1997.

Morrow, John. *History of Political Thought: A Thematic Introduction*. London: Macmillan, 1998.

Mulgan, Richard. "The Processes of Public Accountability." *Australian Journal of Public Administration* 56, 1 (March 1997): 25–36.

Mumford, Lewis. *The Pentagon of Power: The Myth of the Machine*. vol. 2. New York: Harcourt Brace Jovanovich, 1970.

Negri, Antonio, and Michael Hardt. *Empire*. Cambridge, MA: Harvard University Press, 2000.

Neill, Monty. *How the Principles and Indicators for Student Assessment Systems Should Affect Practice*. Cambridge, MA: National Center for Fair and Open Testing, 1996.

Nevitte, Neil. "Value Change and Reorientations in Citizen-State Relations." *Canadian Public Policy* 26 (2000): 73–94.

North, Douglass. *Structure and Change in Economic History*. New York: Norton, 1981.

Nozick, Robert. *Anarchy, State, and Utopia*. New York: Basic Books, 1974.

O'Brien, M. A. Thompson, A. D. Oxman, R. B. Haynes, D. A. Davis, N. Freemantle, and E. L. Harvey. "Local Opinion Leaders: Efforts on Professional Practice and Health Care Outcomes." *Cochrane Review 2001* (Cochrane. Database. Syst. Rev. CD00125).

Ohmae, Kenici. *The End of the Nation-State*. New York: The Free Press, 1995.

Okun, Arthur. *Equality and Efficiency: The Big Trade-Off*. Washington, D.C.: Brookings Institution, 1975.

O'Neill, John. *The Poverty of Postmodernism*. New York: Routledge, 1995.

Osborne, David, and Ted Gaebler. *Reinventing Government*. New York: Plume, 1993.

Paine, Thomas. *Rights of Man*. In *Thomas Paine Reader*, edited by Michael Foot and Isaac Kramnick. New York: Penguin Books, 1987.

Pareto, Vilfredo. *Manual of Political Economy*, translated by Ann S. Schwier and Alfred N. Page. New York: A. M. Kelley, 1971.

Pateman, Carole. *Participation and Democratic Theory*. Cambridge: Cambridge University Press, 1970.

Pauly, Louis W. *Who Elected the Bankers? Surveillance and Control in the World Economy*. Ithaca, NY: Cornell University Press, 1997.

Plato. *The Republic*, edited by A. D. Linsay. London: Dent, 1976.

Pole, Ken. "Canadians Concerned about the Efficiency and Accountability of Care." *The Medical Post* 37, 9 (Mar. 6, 2001).

Priest, Lisa. *Operating in the Dark: Accountability in Our Health Care System*. Toronto: The Atkinson Foundation, 1999.

Putman, Robert. "Tuning In, Tuning Out: The Strange Disappearance of Social Capital in America." *PS: Political Science and Politics*, 28 (1995): 664–83.

Rabinbach, Anson. *The Human Motor: Energy, Fatigue, and the Origins of Modernity*. New York: Basic Books, 1990.

Radwanski, George. *Ontario Study of the Relevance of Education and the Issue of Dropouts*. Toronto: Ontario Ministry of Education, 1987.

Rae, Bob. *The Three Questions: Prosperity and the Public Good*. Toronto: Viking, 1998.

Rappolt, Susan. "Clinical Guidelines and the Fate of Medical Autonomy in Ontario." *Social Science and Medicine* 44, 7 (1997): 977–87.

Rawls, John. *A Theory of Justice*. Cambridge, MA: Harvard University Press, 1971.

Raz, Joseph. *The Morality of Freedom*. Oxford: Clarendon Press, 1986.

Reeve, Andrew. "Individual Choice and the Retreat from Utilitarianism." In *The Utilitarian Response: The Contemporary Viability of Utilitarian Political Philosophy*, edited by Lincoln Allison. London: Jay, 1990.

Reich, Robert B. "The Choice Fetish." *Civilization* 7, 4 (Aug. 2000): 64–66.

Robin, Corey. "The Ex-Cons: Right-Wing Thinkers Go Left!" *Lingua Franca* 11, 1 (Feb. 2001): 24–33.

Rodrik, Dani. "Why Do More Open Economies Have Bigger Governments?" *Journal of Political Economy* (forthcoming 2001).

Rouse, Cecilia. "Private-School Vouchers and Student Achievement. An Evaluation of the Milwaukee Parental Choice Program." *Quarterly Journal of Economics* 113, 2 (May 1998): 553–602.

Ruggie, John. *Winning the Peace: America and World Order in the New Era*. New York: Columbia University Press, 1996.

Sachs, Jeffrey. "International Economics: Unlocking the Mysteries of Globalization." *Foreign Policy* 110 (1998): 97–111.

Saskatchewan Commission on Medicare. *Caring for Medicare: Sustaining a Quality System*. Saskatoon: Saskatchewan Commission on Medicare, 2001.

Saul, John Ralston. *The Unconscious Civilization*. Toronto: Anansi, 1995.

Schiesl, Martin J. *The Politics of Efficiency: Municipal Administration and Reform in America. 1800–1920*. Berkeley: University of California Press, 1977.

Schlesinger, Arthur. *The Imperial Presidency*. Boston: Houghton Mifflin, 1973.

Schneider, Mark. "Institutional Arrangements and the Creation of Social Capital: The Effects of Public School

Choice." *American Political Science Review* 41, 1 (March 1997): 82–93.

Schofield, John. "Saving Our Schools." *Maclean's* (May 14, 2000): 22–29.

Schreyer, Paul. "The OECD Productivity Manual: A Guide to the Measurement of Industry-Level and Aggregate Productivity." *International Productivity Monitor* 2 (Spring 2001): 37–51.

Sen, Amartya. *Development As Freedom*. New York: Knopf, 1999.

———. *Poverty and Famines: An Essay on Entitlement and Deprivation*. Oxford: Clarendon Press, 1982.

———. "Rational Fools: A Critique of the Behavioural Foundations of Economic Theory." *Philosophy and Public Affairs* 6, 4 (1977): 317–44.

Senge, Peter. *The Fifth Discipline: The Art and Practice of the Learning Organization*. New York: Doubleday, 1990.

Shaw, R. Paul. *New Trends in Public-Sector Management in Health: Applications in Developed and Developing Countries*. Washington, D.C.: World Bank Institute, 1999.

Sharpe, Andrew. "Determinants of Trends in Living Standards in Canada and the United States, 1989–2000." *International Productivity Monitor* 2 (Spring 2001): 3–10.

Sheppard, Robert. "We Are Canadian." *Maclean's* 113/114, 1/52 (Dec. 25, 2000/Jan.1, 2001): 26–32.

Shleifer, Andrei, and Robert Vishny. *The Grabbing Hand: Government Pathologies and Their Cures*. Cambridge, MA: Harvard University Press, 1998.

Sidgwick, Henry. *The Elements of Politics*. London: Macmillan, 1891.

Simunovic, Marko, Anna Gagliardi, David McCready, Angela Coates, Mark Levine, and Denny Depatrillo. "A Snapshot of Waiting Times for Cancer Surgery Provided by Surgeons Affiliated with Cancer Centres in

Ontario." *Canadian Medical Association Journal* 165, 4 (Aug. 21, 2001): 421–25.

Smilie, Ian. "NGOs and Development Assistance: A Change in Mind-set?" *Third World Quarterly* 18, 3 (1997): 563–77.

Smith, Adam. *An Inquiry into the Nature and Causes of the Wealth of Nations*, edited by R. H. Campbell and A. S. Skinner. Oxford: Clarendon Press, 1975.

———. *Theory of Moral Sentiments*, edited by D. D. Raphael and A. L. Macfie. Oxford: Clarendon Press, 1976.

———. *The Wealth of Nations*, edited by A. Skinner. Harmondsworth: Penguin Classics, 1981.

Smith, James Allen. *The Idea Brokers*. New York: The Free Press, 1991.

Stein, Janice Gross, Richard Stren, Joy Fitzgibbon, and Melissa MacLean. *Networks of Knowledge: Collaborative Innovation in International Learning*. Toronto: University of Toronto Press, 2001.

Stevenson, Harold. "A TIMSS Primer." *Fordham Report* 2, 7 (1998), pp. 1–28.

Stone, Deborah. *Policy Paradox and Political Reason*. New York: HarperCollins, 1988.

Strange, Susan. *The Retreat of the State: The Diffusion of Power in the World Economy*. Cambridge: Cambridge University Press, 1996.

Taylor, Frederick Winslow. *The Principles of Scientific Management*. New York: Harper and Bros., 1911. Reprint, 1947.

Thompson, Thomas. "State of the State Address" (Madison, W.I., January 1995).

Tilly, Charles. "Reflections on the History of European State-Making." In *The Formation of National States in Western Europe*, edited by Charles Tilly. Princeton, NJ: Princeton University Press, 1975.

Trebilcock, Michael. *The Prospects for Reinventing*

Government. Toronto: C. D. Howe Institute, 1994.

Trebilcock, Michael, Ron Daniels, and Michael Thorburn. "Government by Voucher." *Boston University Law Review* 80 (2000): 205–32.

Tullock, Gordon. *Private Wants, Public Means: An Economic Analysis of the Desirable Scope of Government*. New York: Basic Books, 1970.

Tuohy, Carolyn. *Accidental Logics: The Dynamics of Change in the Health Care Arena in the United States, Britain, and Canada*. New York: Oxford University Press, 1999.

Tuohy, Carolyn, Colleen Flood, and Mark Stabile. *How Does Private Finance Affect Public Health Care Systems?* Toronto: University of Toronto working paper, 2001.

Tyack, David B. *The One Best System: A History of American Urban Education*. Cambridge, MA: Harvard University Press, 1974.

Van den Berg, Axel. "Politics versus Markets: A Note on the Uses of Double Standards." Paper presented to Reinventing Society in a Changing Global Economy Conference. University of Toronto, March 8–9, 2001.

Van den Berg, Axel, and Joseph Smucker, eds. *The Sociology of Labour Markets: Efficiency, Equity, Security*. Toronto: Prentice-Hall Canada, 1997.

Warrian, Peter. "From Industrywide Bargaining to Individuation: Changing Social Values of Local Union Leaders." Unpublished paper, Toronto, April 2001.

———. *Hard Bargain: Transforming Public-Sector Labour-Management Relations*. Toronto: McGilligan Books, 1996.

Weber, Max. "Politics As a Vocation." In *From Max Weber*, edited by H. H. Gerth and C. W. Mills. New York: Oxford University Press, 1972.

Wildavsky, Aaron. *Speaking Truth to Power: The Art and Craft of Policy Analysis*. Boston: Little Brown, 1979.

Wilkinson, Richard G. *Unhealthy Societies: The Afflictions of Inequality*. London: Routledge, 1996.

Witte, John F. *The Market Approach to Education: An Analysis of America's First Voucher Program*. Princeton, NJ: Princeton University Press, 2000.

Wolfe, Alan. "The Final Freedom." *New York Times Magazine* (Mar. 18, 2001): 48–51.

Xenophon. *History of Greece* 1.7. In *Democracy: Ideas and Realities*, edited by C. Rodewald. London: Dent, 1974.

Zacher, Mark. "The Global Economy and the International Political Order." In *The Nation State in a Global/Information Era: Policy Challenges*, edited by Thomas Courchene. Kingston: John Deutsch Institute for Economic Research, 1999.

Zolo, Danilo. *Democracy and Complexity*, translated by David McKie. Cambridge: Polity Press, 1992.